Recent Advances in
GERIATRIC MEDICINE

BERNARD ISAACS MD FRCP (Glas) MRCP (Edin)
Charles Hayward Professor of Geriatric Medicine
University of Birmingham

Recent Advances in GERIATRIC MEDICINE

EDITED BY

BERNARD ISAACS

NUMBER ONE

CHURCHILL LIVINGSTONE
EDINBURGH LONDON AND NEW YORK 1978

CHURCHILL LIVINGSTONE
Medical Division of Longman Group Limited

Distributed in the United States of America by Longman Inc., 19 West 44th Street, New York, N.Y. 10036 and by associated companies, branches and representatives throughout the world

First published 1978

ISBN 0 443 01519 8

British Library Cataloguing in Publication Data
Recent advances in geriatric medicine.
No. 1
1 Geriatrics
I. Isaacs, Bernard, b. 1924
618.9'7 RC952 77-30316

Printed in Great Britain by Adlard & Son Ltd, Bartholomew Press, Dorking

Preface

Textbooks and monographs on geriatric medicine have been appearing in a steady stream in recent years, while a wide range of general and specialist journals have published a growing body of research work. The invitation to devote a volume of the well-established Recent Advances series to geriatric medicine is an encouraging indication of the growing professional interest in the medicine of late life and of the need that is now being felt to bring new knowledge before a wider audience of general and specialist readers.

Virtually all doctors practise the medicine of old age; but in the United Kingdom the specialty of geriatric medicine has developed distinctively. Consultant physicians devoting their full time to the practice of medicine in the elderly have stood at the growing points of knowledge. As a reflection of this unique British system all the contributors to this volume come from the United Kingdom. Many are full-time physicians in geriatric medicine, and many of the advances recorded here are their work. Other contributors come from a variety of disciplines, and their interest in the elderly has been stimulated by their awareness of the needs of this group and of the burning scientific questions that they pose.

The editor wishes to combine his thanks to the team of contributors with his expression of regret that there was no space to cull more widely from the many topics where advances have occurred and from the many authors who have contributed to these. A final word of thanks is due to Sue Trobridge and Valerie Kedge for their assistance in the preparation of the manuscript.

Birmingham 1977

Bernard Isaacs

Contributors

A. J. AKHTAR MB BSc FRCP
Consultant in Geriatric Medicine, Royal Victoria Hospital, Edinburgh; and part-time Senior Lecturer, Department of Geriatric Medicine, University of Edinburgh

SIR FERGUSON ANDERSON OBE KStJ MD FRCP(Glas Lond Edin) FRCPI FRCPC
David Cargill Professor of Geriatric Medicine, University of Glasgow, Stobhill General Hospital, Glasgow

JOHN CHARLES BROCKLEHURST MSc MD FRCP (Edin Glas)
Professor of Geriatric Medicine, University of Manchester, University Hospital of South Manchester, Manchester

DAVID M. BOWEN PhD
Senior Lecturer in Neurochemistry, Miriam Marks Department of Neurochemistry, The National Hospital, London

ALAN N. DAVISON BPharm PhD DSc
Professor of Neurochemistry, Miriam Marks Department of Neurochemistry, The National Hospital, London

A. N. EXTON-SMITH MD FRCP
Barlow Professor of Geriatric Medicine, University College Hospital Medical School, London

W. M. GARRAWAY MB MSc MFCM
Lecturer, Department of Community Medicine, University of Edinburgh

COLIN GODBER MRCP MRCPsych MPhil
Consultant Psychogeriatrician, Moorgreen Hospital, Southampton

M. R. P. HALL BM FRCP (Lond Edin)
Professor of Geriatric Medicine, University of Southampton

I. R. HASTIE MB MRCP
Lecturer in Geriatric Medicine, St George's Hospital, London

H. M. HODKINSON MA DM FRCP
Consultant Physician in Geriatric Medicine, Northwick Park Hospital, Harrow, Middlesex

P. H. MILLARD MB FRCP
Consultant Physician and Senior Lecturer in Geriatric Medicine, St George's Hospital, London

P. W. OVERSTALL MB MRCP
Consultant Physician in Geriatric Medicine, University College Hospital, St Pancras Hospital, London

C. P. SILVER DM FRCP
Consultant Geriatrician, The London Hospital

JAMES WILLIAMSON MB ChB FRCP(Edin)
Professor of Geriatric Medicine, University of Edinburgh, City Hospital, Edinburgh

Contents

Has geriatric medicine advanced?

Bernard Isaacs

Has geriatric medicine advanced? Has it even justified itself as a specialty? What indeed is geriatric medicine, and what constitutes a 'recent advance' in that subject? These and related questions are discussed in this chapter.

Definition of geriatric medicine

Definitions of geriatric medicine comprise those written by geriatricians, which describe what they wish to do for their elderly patients; and those written by non-geriatricians, which describe what they wish to have done for theirs. Geriatricians are specialists, trained in general (internal) medicine, with three additional attributes—commitment to the elderly; the jealous guarding of professional standards; and awareness of what has been done in their field by those who went before. The varied practices of geriatric medicine result from the varied patterns of interaction between the geriatric physician, his resources and his colleagues in medical, paramedical and social fields.

What are 'advances' in geriatric medicine?

Advances in geriatric medicine consist of new knowledge which directly or indirectly benefits ill old people. Advances come from geriatricians, non-geriatricians and from collaboration between the two. The advances comprise:

1. Studies of clinical syndromes which occur largely or exclusively in the elderly; or which present distinctive characteristics in old age; or which require special treatment in old people.
2. Studies of relation between clinical, laboratory and pathological processes in old age.
3. Studies of the medical and social characteristics of elderly populations; their 'normal' attributes; the prevalence and distribution of diseases and disability; and changes in these features with time.
4. Operational studies of the methods and resources required for the prevention and relief of disease and disability in the elderly.
5. Design and evaluation of the equipment and the environment designed for the treatment of disease and the management of disability.
6. Education of health professionals and of the general public in the features of health and illness in later life.
7. Formulation of the concepts of geriatric medicine.

Advances in the understanding of the biological processes of ageing, which are of great potential importance, are not included here under the heading of advances in geriatric medicine.

Formulation of concepts

The day-to-day decisions of doctors in most fields of medicine are based on assumptions which are seldom questioned. Examples of these are:

1. There is a clear differentiation between 'health' and 'disease'.
2. Diseases exist as separate entities.
3. Disease can be recognised by clinical and laboratory study.
4. Precise diagnosis precedes treatment.
5. Patients offer a frank and accurate account of their symptoms.
6. Treatment is beneficial.
7. Treatment is desired.
8. The objectives of treatment can be stated.
9. The attainment of these objectives can be recognised.
10. Treatment is not restrained by shortage of resources.

Few, if any, of these assumptions can be made confidently in geriatric medicine. In old age pathological changes are rife in cells, tissues and organs; every gradation is found between 'health' and 'disease'; 'illness' represents the impaired function of many organs; 'improvement in the quality of life' rather than restoration of normality becomes the objective of medical intervention. Treatment does not await total diagnosis; amelioration is sought rather than cure; denial of illness often makes treatment unacceptable; prolongation of life is not necessarily seen as a desirable end in itself. Resources do not stretch to the invariable prescription of optimum treatment.

These considerations place the geriatric physician in a distinctive relation to his patient, and give new importance to once-familiar but long-unexplored issues. For example, the ability to define the 'normal' becomes a matter neither of semantics nor of statistics, but a burning issue to be decided afresh at every clinical intervention. The failure to define normality makes victims alike of the elderly patient whose distressing symptoms of disease are dismissed as 'normal for his age', and the symptomless old person whose aberrant biochemical or physiological findings cause him to be subjected to irrelevant investigation or hazardous medication.

Advances in the formulation of concepts are translated into advances in the treatment of patients and are thus, no less than the more spectacular developments in ward and laboratory, truly advances in geriatric medicine.

Hypertension in old age

The argument is illustrated by considering the issues which underlie an everyday and apparently simple question, namely, when should raised blood pressure in the elderly be treated?

A few of the many subsidiary questions to which this gives rise will be considered:

1. Who are the elderly?
2. What is raised blood pressure?
3. What is the object of treatment?
4. What are the resource implications of treatment?

Who are the elderly?

The 'elderly', comprising many millions of the population of Western countries, are too often referred to as though they were a homogeneous group. A minimal subdivision for the clarification of medical questions is into six age-and-sex groups, i.e. those of each sex in the age groups 65 to 74, 75 to 84 and 85 and over, respectively.

An alternative grouping might be into those of each sex who have and who have not attained their average life expectancy, i.e. men aged 65 to 69; men aged 70 and over; women aged 65 to 74; and women aged 75 and over.

The significance of a clinical finding in an old person very much depends on which group he belongs to. Rarely can data be found which give separate guidance on the significance of a clinical finding or on the expectation of life of a given disease in each of these age and sex groups.

THE VERY OLD

Very old people differ from those who are their juniors by 10 or 20 years in several important ways:

1. The very old, by virtue of having been born before the less old, were exposed to different environmental factors in their earlier life, such as diet, atmospheric pollution, working conditions. They received less education, earned less money, had larger families and developed different social expectations.
2. Old people are the survivors. Those aged 65 represent two-thirds of their birth-cohort; those aged 75 one-half; and those aged 85 one-tenth of theirs.
3. Time-related changes in the cells, organs and tissues have had longer to operate in the very old.
4. The very old comprise those who have survived because they have sustained little pathological change; those who have survived despite having sustained much pathological change; and every gradation between.

SAMPLING

Concepts of the 'normal' in younger people are derived from random samples of the healthy population. The difficulties of sampling increase with age, in regard both to the criteria of 'healthy' and the practicalities of recruitment. Many statements about the 'normal' are derived from selected groups, e.g. the residents of old people's homes; or highly motivated professional people.

What is raised blood pressure?

Setting aside such technical questions as how was the blood pressure recorded, in what body position, at what time of day, and how often, a given reading may be deemed to be 'raised' in one of four ways, i.e. as compared with:

1. The mean and standard deviation of readings taken from a population of healthy adults.
2. The mean and standard deviation of readings taken from a general population sample of the same age and sex as the patient.
3. Readings obtained from the same patient at an earlier stage of his life.
4. The demonstration of a rate of change in the individual which exceeds the normal rate of change.

While information has been collected about the mean and standard deviation of casual and resting systolic and diastolic blood pressure in populations of old people, there is much doubt about how this should be related to a reading in a given elderly patient. Normal values for blood pressure in healthy young adult populations do not necessarily define normal or raised blood pressure in old age. Differences in different epochs make it desirable to renew frequently basic population studies. Within these limitations a blood pressure reading in an old person probably can be characterised as 'raised' in relation to the mean for his age and sex group.

Data about rises in the blood pressure of the individual are difficult to validate unless a record exists of the circumstances in which previous readings were obtained. Clear evidence of a rise over a period of time must be compared with the experience of the population, and there are few, if any, studies of changes in blood pressure over time which would allow the question of whether a given rise is greater than the rise for the population as a whole to be answered.

The question 'What is raised blood pressure in the elderly?' might thus comprise four separate questions in each of four or six age-and-sex groups. The area of uncertainty is large.

What is the object of treatment?

High blood pressure in younger people is a cause of morbidity and premature death, especially from heart disease and stroke. In such young people the treatment of symptomless hypertension is justified. In older people the questions need to be asked afresh. Are symptomless old people at the same type of risk as younger ones? If so, the benefits of treatment have to be established quantitatively so that decisions can be made on the prophylactic value of antihypertensive treatment in groups of old people.

In patients with symptoms attributable to hypertension the matter is fortunately simple. The symptoms of hypertensive heart disease can be treated by diuretic drugs which have a hypotensive effect, i.e. thiazides; and treatment with specific antihypertensive drugs may not be necessary. Treatment is maintained indefinitely, since its withdrawal produces relapse of the heart failure.

The side-effects of antihypertensive drugs most feared in the elderly are hypokalaemia and postural hypotension. One adverse experience of weakness, dizziness or falls, frightens the patient and destroys his compliance. Often treatment is not maintained with sufficient thoroughness to determine its effectiveness. Even in the absence of side-effects the accuracy with which old people take drugs is highly suspect. Patients who live alone, those with memory defect, those unable to read labels or to open bottles, those with difficulty in swallowing and those on multiple medication are especially likely to lapse in their drug taking.

Resource implications

Once a doctor decides to treat an elderly symptomless patient with high blood pressure by antihypertensive drugs he is obliged to organise a monitoring system. The fortunate British general practitioner, with a fixed list of patients, can draw up his age–sex register to identify the patients whom he proposes to survey. These will be approached by a health visitor, tested, sent for medical examination, prescribed and monitored. All such series suffer high losses, and the conclusions drawn from the persevering minority cannot be applied to the lapsed. Clear answers to questions are unlikely to come from small-scale trials based on the experience of individual doctors, while the benefit to be obtained from large-scale studies may not seem to be sufficient to justify their expense.

Ethical issues

Sociologists complain that old people are deprived of their freedom of choice. The administration of antihypertensive drugs affects several aspects of the old person's life. The possible advantage that the risk of stroke or heart attack may be reduced and useful life prolonged by a year or two is to be weighed against the disadvantages of involvement with doctor and health visitor, the need to remember to take medicine daily and the risk of suffering dizzy attacks or falling. Should these issues be presented to the patient in a way in which he can understand and should the choice be his? Or is it better for the patient's sake to preserve his confidence in the infallibility of the doctor by making the decision for him? A developing area of research is that which contrasts the doctor's view of the patient with the patient's view of the doctor.

The balance of benefit

The question 'When should old people take antihypertensive drugs?' illustrates the complexity of clinical problems in geriatric medicine, the wide areas of uncertainty, the elusiveness of clarification. Similar conceptual issues underlie many other practical questions that are encountered daily in geriatric medicine, such as: what significance should be attached to the finding of glycosuria or of a raised alkaline phosphatase or a systolic murmur or a goitre? The research issues cover a wide range from epidemiology to diagnostic, therapeutic and operational problems. Fortunately, doctors are accustomed to treating patients by the 'art of medicine' without awaiting research results. Geriatric medicine, too, has its artistry; but the type of research indicated here, based on clarification of complex processes, will provide the doctor with guidance. In the meantime elderly patients with high blood pressure will be treated by doctors who are sensitive to the balance of benefit which forms the background to decision-making in geriatric medicine.

1. Theory and practice of stroke rehabilitation

Michael Garraway   Anwar J. Akhtar

INTRODUCTION

It has been suggested by a recent report from the World Health Organisation (1971) that no single measure could so improve the quality of life in old people as the prevention of stroke. Information on some of the predisposing factors contributing to stroke has been obtained over the past 25 years (Kannel et al, 1965, 1967, 1970, 1974; Kurtzke 1969; American Heart Association, 1971). Although specific efforts at prevention by primary or secondary intervention have been made in ischaemic heart disease, little effort has been directed towards stroke. Recent published evidence on hypertension, one of the predisposing factors, suggests that a potential reduction in incidence might be possible (US Veterans' Administration Study Group 1967, 1970, 1972). Stroke prevention can be regarded as in its infancy, and considerable resources will have to be devoted to stroke rehabilitation in the coming decades.

DEFINITION OF STROKE

'Stroke' can be defined as the sudden onset of a focal neurological deficit due to a local disturbance in blood supply to the brain. 'Sudden' refers to a time period which may range from a few seconds to several hours or even several days (World Health Organisation, 1971). The underlying vascular disturbance, whether it is stenotic, occlusive or rupture of an intra- or extracerebral artery, manifests itself as various neurological symptoms. These are related to the extent and site of the area involved, to the speed with which the pathological process develops, and to the underlying condition. The neurological manifestations in turn produce physical and/or mental impairment, leading to transient or permanent disability and handicap.

REHABILITATION

To counteract the effect of residual impairment following stroke and to minimise handicap require the application of rehabilitation, which was defined by the World Health Organisation (1969) as 'the combined and coordinated use of medical, social, educational and vocational measures for training or retraining the individual to the highest possible level of functional ability'.

This chapter deals with the background to stroke rehabilitation; aspects of the practice of stroke rehabilitation; and some of the growing points in the field.

Neurological background

Stroke is a vascular lesion which presents with neurological manifestations. These can be many and varied, according to the site, extent, type, spread and speed with which the vascular lesion becomes established. A comprehensive account of the historical aspects of stroke and the development of its rehabilitation has been published by Licht (1975); while the pathological basis of cerebrovascular disease has been dealt with elsewhere (Brocklehurst, 1973).

There are remarkable variations in the neurological manifestations of stroke, ranging from an abrupt onset and rapid evolution of hemiplegia with loss of consciousness to a slow cumulative change in the neurological picture over months or even years. This may consist only of some slight deficit or derangement of speech, thought or voluntary movement, with no change in conscious level. The neurological manifestations of stroke may last for seconds, minutes or longer, or they may persist indefinitely. Even once neurological manifestations are established they do not remain static, and some improvement in neurological impairment almost always occurs amongst stroke survivors. In addition to the 'focal neurological deficit' implicit in the definition of stroke, which may be manifest as signs such as homonymous hemianopia, there may be a more diffuse or general disturbance of neurological function. For example, symptoms such as drowsiness or confusion which cannot be attributed to a particular anatomical region of the brain may be present. These diffuse neurological manifestations produced by the underlying vascular insult to the brain are usually transient and more reversible than the focal signs and symptoms.

The variety of stroke presentation is further complicated by other clinical features which may or may not be related to the underlying pathogenesis of cerebrovascular disease. The entire constellation of clinical features must be taken into account. For example, there may be hypertension or diabetes, or a source of emboli such as atrial fibrillation or evidence of vascular disease at other sites such as the heart or lower limbs.

A useful classification of the neurological manifestations of stroke based on clinical experience has been suggested by Isaacs (1973) and a detailed summary of the clinical presentations of the principal types of cerebrovascular disease was produced some years ago (Advisory Council for the National Institute of Neurological Diseases and Blindness, 1958).

Epidemiological background

A considerable amount of effort has been put into quantifying the frequency and distribution of stroke. The United Kingdom comes high up in the stroke mortality league table. Scotland has a higher overall age-adjusted death rate than England and Wales, and Northern Ireland, and has the highest age-adjusted mortality rate from cerebrovascular disease of all the members of the European Economic Community (World Health Organisation, 1975).

Cerebrovascular disease is the third commonest cause of death in Scotland, accounting for 15.71 per cent of all deaths in 1975 (Registrar General for Scotland, 1977). This is exceeded only by ischaemic heart disease and malignant neoplasms as in many other developed countries. Age-specific death rates for cerebrovascular disease in Scotland roughly treble through each decade of life. Reservations have been expressed about the validity of mortality data which ascribes the cause of death to cerebrovascular disease (Heasman and Lipworth, 1966). When this fact is allied to an autopsy rate of only 4.2 per cent of cerebrovascular disease deaths occurring at home, and only 14.3 per cent of such deaths occurring in hospital (Registrar General for Scotland, 1976), one can see that mortality statistics do not take us very far towards understanding the clinical picture of stroke.

Studies of stroke morbidity provide a more accurate assessment of the size of the problem. Two carefully conducted studies from the Mayo Clinic (Whisnant et al, 1971; Matsumoto et al, 1973) can be chosen from many published in the past 15 years that have estimated the incidence, i.e. the number of new cases of stroke occurring in a given population during a given period of time and the prevalence, i.e. the number of strokes in a defined population at a particular point in time (point prevalence) or in a stated period of time (period prevalence). The incidence of stroke was estimated to be 1.64/1000 of population per annum, with a period prevalence of 5.97 strokes/1000 population per annum.

There is a dramatic increase in stroke morbidity with age. Cerebral infarction, including emboli, accounted for 79 per cent of all strokes in the Mayo Clinic series; cerebral haemorrhage for 10 per cent; and subarachnoid haemorrhage for 6 per cent.

Up to 50 per cent of the mortality which results from stroke occurs in the first three weeks following onset (Eisenberg et al, 1964). Once this initial period of high mortality is over, the prognosis for life in stroke is comparatively good, with a constant probability of dying of approximately 8 per cent per annum. This, it has been postulated, is because the risk of dying for survivors of the immediate period of mortality is related not to the mental or physical disability caused by the lesion but to the slow progression of the underlying vascular disease (Marquardsen, 1969). Thus the natural history of stroke follows a pattern similar to that of acute myocardial infarction, with a high period of early mortality and then a good prognosis for life for the survivors. However, unlike survivors of myocardial infarction, who regain independence in weeks or months (Sharland, 1964) stroke survivors have high levels of physical and mental dependency as a result of residual disability.

CONSEQUENCES OF STROKE

The pattern of the natural history of cerebrovascular disease, together with the neurological and associated impairments which produce residual mental and physical disability, have consequences for the individual stroke patient who is handicapped, and for the resources of health and social services utilised to support stroke patients. These factors have an important bearing on the aims of stroke rehabilitation and on the organisation and distribution of resources.

Functional disability

The residual effect of stroke is the disability which remains after maximal clinical and functional recovery has taken place. Precise knowledge of this long-term disability is important as a prognostic index. In a number of studies groups of stroke patients have been followed and their residual disability estimated. Although each series of patients was assessed using different criteria of functional impairment, a broad consensus can be seen in the results. For example, in the Fredericksberg series (Marquardsen, 1969) 404 patients who were admitted to a neurological unit survived the early period of high mortality and were subsequently rehabilitated. Five per cent of these died in hospital within two months; 16 per cent were able to carry out all their normal activities at the time of discharge from hospital; 52 per cent had disability which required some help with self-care; and 27 per cent could not undertake any self-care unaided, or required constant attention.

The data is based on a selected group of stroke patients admitted to hospital, and emphasises the low proportion of stroke survivors who regain complete independence. It is seldom possible to distinguish with confidence potential levels of residual disability in stroke patients before 10 to 12 weeks. Patients may continue to improve up to 12 or even

18 months after the onset of a stroke (Hurwitz and Adams, 1972). This does not appear to exert much influence on the distribution of disability at a later stage. Rankin (1957) found that only 19 per cent of survivors in a series of 252 patients admitted to hospital in Glasgow were able to carry out all their usual activities six months after the onset of a stroke. Of 119 stroke patients followed up for a mean period of seven years in Framingham (Gresham et al, 1975) only 29 per cent had no loss of vocational function, i.e. had returned to work or homemaking activities; and 30 per cent had normal socialisation outside the home. Twenty per cent of patients were dependent for mobility and 31 per cent for activities of daily living. Only 10 per cent of patients had no discernible functional deficit. Thus a reservoir of disability is created by strokes, which will increase every year as large cohorts of people projected to enter old age in the coming decades are afflicted by stroke. It has been estimated that there are 130 000 persons in private households in Great Britain who are handicapped by stroke (Harris, 1971). Thirty per cent of such persons are in need of special care, being dependent on someone else for the performance of daily living activities. This expanding reservoir of disability has important implications for the utilisation of resources within the National Health Service, and, in particular, for the distribution of rehabilitation resources.

Burden on resources

Despite the size of the reservoir of stroke in the community, the real impact on resources is made in the hospital service. Cerebrovascular disease is a leading cause of hospital admission in Scotland, comprising 2.6 per cent of all admissions in 1973, excluding maternity and mental illness. The proportion of beds utilised by patients with cerebrovascular disease is much higher. In 1973 cerebrovascular disease accounted for the highest occupancy of hospital bed days in Scotland of any single disease group, using 1 076 254 bed-days, which represents 11.2 per cent of all bed-days in all specialties in that year, excluding mental illness and maternity. If population projections are accurate, if the criteria for hospital admission remain the same, and if the number of available bed-days remains constant, patients with cerebrovascular disease will occupy 17.3 per cent of bed-days in 1991, excluding mental illness and maternity. This represents an increase of 65 per cent over the utilisation of beds by patients with cerebrovascular disease in 1973. These beds are predominantly occupied by elderly patients; less than 10 per cent in 1973 being under 65 years of age (Scottish Hospital In-patient Statistics, 1975). Sixty-five per cent of stroke patients were admitted as emergencies, general medical units making by far the largest contribution in receiving 56 per cent of all stroke admissions.

PRINCIPLES OF STROKE REHABILITATION

Given that stroke is one of the major caring problems created by any single disease group, what is the optimum level of resources to be devoted to the rehabilitation of stroke? Where should these resources be located? How should rehabilitation be conducted and which stroke patients derive benefit from rehabilitation?

The concept of rehabilitation is relatively unfamiliar to a large section of the medical profession (Occupational Therapy, 1974), partly because of its absence from the undergraduate curriculum of most, if not all, medical schools. Wylie (1974) found that the attitude of general practitioners to stroke rehabilitation depended in part on the undergraduate education; and doctors from one particular medical school were singularly disinterested in stroke patients and their rehabilitation. He concluded that improved undergraduate teaching of rehabilitation would appear to be the long-term remedy. Of all diseases leading to chronic disability, stroke, more than any other, gives rise to feelings of dejection and helplessness in the medical attendant. The outlook for the stroke patient was exceedingly poor till quite recently (Adams, 1971; Lowman, 1948). He was relegated to some shadowy corner of the ward beyond the natural gaze of the attendant doctor, in the hope that he would die. In recent years there has been a small-scale shift of emphasis from academic neurology and the localisation of lesions, to the appraisal of neurological deficits which predict the likelihood of functional recovery. This approach allows doctors to communicate intelligently with members of the rehabilitation disciplines and to assist in the allocation of scarce specialist rehabilitation time. The application of this approach has resulted in the creation of multidisciplinary teams for the rehabilitation of stroke, in which the medical contribution is no longer remote from the practical problems presented by the patient's disabilities.

Before treatment is started the patient must be assessed by the different disciplines involved, so that a programme of rehabilitation appropriate to his capacity and requirements may be worked out (Hewer, 1976). Six criteria of assessment have been described (Adams, 1974) and these will be considered in greater detail later on. Rehabilitation should begin as early as possible after a stroke (Steinman, 1976; Anderson, 1966), delay in seeking rehabilitation being associated with high disability (Wylie, 1960).

Passive movements of all limbs on the affected side may be started during the acute phase (Nichols, 1976) even if the patient is unconscious. The importance of being gentle with the paralysed arm during this phase has been stressed. A hemiplegic must never be moved by one nurse unaided lest permanent damage is done to the shoulder joint on the affected side (Nichols, 1976). The physician in geriatric medicine is likely to encounter the patient when he is fully conscious and the neurological deficit has ceased to progress. At this stage the facilities of the rehabilitation unit are of greatest value.

Because of the scarcity of rehabilitation time, it is usually necessary to exclude some patients from intensive treatment. Selection may result in patients being denied treatment who would otherwise make better use of their recovery (Hurwitz, and Adams, 1972; Adams, 1971). Pre-stroke physical or mental disability severe enough to deny the patient independence, is perhaps the only reliable indicator of a poor functional prognosis, no matter how intensively or for how long the patient is subjected to rehabilitation (Adams, 1971). In most patients, rehabilitation must be continued for at least 16 weeks (Adams, 1971) before lack of improvement is taken to indicate a poor prognosis and to raise the possibility of permanent residence in hospital.

PROGNOSIS IN STROKE

Until recent years prognosis after a stroke was considered in terms of the survival or death of the patient. A major advance has been to emphasise the importance of neurological deficits that adversely affect functional recovery and present barriers to successful rehabilitation. The work of Allison in Belfast drew attention to the importance of spatial and perceptual disorders in organic brain disease (Allison, 1962). Adams and Hurwitz in Belfast and Isaacs in Glasgow applied the pioneering approach of Allison to the problem of stroke disability, and thus revolutionised the assessment of the stroke patient (Adams and Hurwitz, 1963; Isaacs, 1971). The criteria of prognostic importance in patients with an established stroke described by Adams (1974) are:

1. Exercise tolerance
2. Motivation
3. Sensory deficit
4. Mental capacity
5. Motor deficit
6. Postural control

Exercise tolerance

This is the endurance of the patient, lack of which prevents him from participating in energetic rehabilitation. Cardiovascular (Peszczynski, 1961) or respiratory disease or physical disability due to rheumatoid arthritis, leg amputation or other chronic condition may seriously tax the patient's endurance, making recovery much less likely. Changes in respiratory function due to the stroke itself, may increase the patient's fatiguability (Hass et al, 1967).

Motivation

This has to do with the will to recover and the capacity to persevere with the task of overcoming disability over many months or years. The ability to apply oneself to simple everyday activities that are no longer effortlessly performed, is essential to motivation. The work of Isaacs has done much to simplify the assessment of these attributes by the use of toys (Isaacs, 1963). The approach of the patient and the way in which he tackles the problem are no less important than ultimate success or failure.

Sensory deficit

Motor weakness due to a stroke has traditionally overshadowed sensory or perceptual abnormalities. This was due, at least in part, to paralysis being more spectacular than defects of sensation or spatial orientation. Also, patients with defective perception seldom draw attention to the peculiar symptoms this may produce, or may even be unaware of its existence. Some disorders of perception, for example, anosognosia or the denial of disease, were considered to be interesting and esoteric and inspired controversy as to their aetiology and significance (Critchley, 1955) but were not considered to be commonplace. The observations of Ullman in the United States (Ullman, 1962) and those of Adams and Hurwitz, and Isaacs (Adams and Hurwitz, 1963; Isaacs and Marks, 1973) in the United Kingdom have done much to increase the awareness of the existence of these remarkably common disorders. The critical importance of defects of proprioception and disorders of spatial orientation leading to neglect of the left half of external space, in patients suffering from stroke, have been emphasised in recent years (Adams, 1974; Isaacs, 1963; Gersten, 1967). Loss of discriminative or cortical sensation is thought to contribute to abnormal movement of the arm and hand; and sensory extinction probably plays some part in the causation of dyspraxia (Adams, 1974). The poor prognosis that accompanies gross and persistent sensory defects is now well established, and tests for their recognition have been described (Isaacs, 1963; Gregory and Aitken, 1971).

Mental capacity

In recent years the critical prognostic importance of mental function after a stroke has been recognised. The classical researches of Adams and Hurwitz mark a turning point in our understanding of the problems of hemiplegia (Adams and Hurwitz, 1963). What appeared to be a mysterious lack of improvement in stroke patients with little or no paralysis, was found by these investigators to be due to defective mental function, producing barriers to recovery. In the 45 long-stay hemiplegic patients investigated by them, about one-half were suffering from a defect of mentation.

Adams and Hurwitz described four mental barriers to recovery. These are of fundamental importance to the understanding of post-stroke behaviour and the patient's response to rehabilitation. In some, defective comprehension of spoken speech seriously interfered with treatment by making communication difficult. The disuse of hemiplegic limbs, denial of disease, denial of ownership of a limb and loss of appreciation of the normal relationship between different parts of the body were responsible for lack of progress in others. 'Space blindness', i.e. the defective localisation of objects in space; apraxia; perseveration; loss of recent memory; emotional lability; and catastrophic reactions were all found in these patients and adversely affected recovery. Adams and Hurwitz emphasised the importance of recognising these disorders as early as possible, 'if mental contractures as rigid as those that develop in neglected paralysed muscles are to be avoided'.

Traditional, elaborate and comprehensive tests of mental function are seldom of value in old people, especially in those who are brain-damaged. They tire quickly, become irritable and lose interest. If they are pressed to co-operate by an enthusiastic investigator, their replies become increasingly unreliable. Several simple clinical tests of mental function give useful information in brain-damaged patients (Ullman, 1962; Allison, 1962; Isaacs and Walkey, 1963; Adams and Hurwitz, 1963; Isaacs and Akhtar, 1972; Milne et al 1972; Hodkinson, 1972; Silver, 1972). The ability to maintain motor activity, for example, protruding the tongue or lateral gaze, has been used to assess brain damage (Ben-Yishay et al, 1968).

Motor deficit

Muscular paralysis and its recovery after stroke have been remarkably little investigated since they were first studied in detail many years ago (Twitchell, 1951; Buskirk, 1954). The degree of weakness correlates highly with the prospect of functional recovery (Gersten, 1975), and absence of spontaneous recovery of power in the affected leg many months after the stroke makes recovery of independence unlikely. There are, however, wide variations in the speed and extent of recovery in paralysed limbs, and voluntary movement may begin to return six months or more after the stroke (Adams, 1974).

Postural control

This is a delicately balanced mechanism of great complexity. An insult to the central nervous system due to a stroke often impairs postural control and balance. The development of spasticity is partly responsible but cannot account for the persistence of this disturbance in the face of prolonged rehabilitation (Adams, 1974). No in-depth research has been done into disordered postural control after a stroke, and descriptions in the literature are mostly based on clinical observations. The work of Purdon Martin into extrapyramidal dysfunction (Martin, 1967) offers a possible model for research into disordered postural control after a stroke.

SOCIAL ASPECTS OF STROKE REHABILITATION

The devastating impact of a stroke on the family is well recognised, but how best to prepare the victim and relatives to cope with the social isolation imposed upon them by this disease, remains a relatively untapped area for investigation. The report of the Royal College of Physicians on strokes (Royal College of Physicians, 1974) outlines some of the deficiencies in services available to stroke patients and their relatives and comments on the lack of interest in their welfare. The education of the family by a multidisciplinary team of professionals who are familiar with their problems has been stressed (*British Medical Journal*, 1974; Overs et al, 1966). The preparation of the family for an unfamiliar lifestyle which may continue for many months or years, and which may require the caring relatives to assume a variety of skilled roles including those of nurse, physiotherapist, psychologist and speech therapist, should commence while the patient is still in hospital (Hurwitz and Adams, 1972). After discharge the primary care team must assume responsibility for continuing support and education.

STROKE REHABILITATION UNITS

The growth of geriatric medicine has highlighted deficiences in the management of surviving stroke patients. There is general agreement that stroke intensive care units, akin to coronary care units, do not reduce the early high mortality (Kennedy et al, 1970). There is some evidence, however, that intensive care reduces the number of complications amongst survivors (Drake et al, 1973). Dispute has arisen on whether stroke units can provide more effective rehabilitation of the survivors. Departments of general medicine, with their emphasis on the investigation and 'cure' of disease, are not equipped in staff or facilities to handle the 'care' problems and the detailed planning required for the rehabilitation of strokes. This has been recognised by the report of a working party of the Royal College of Physicians (1974) which recommended that some departments of geriatric medicine or neurology should develop stroke units. This approach to stroke rehabilitation has already been implemented in a few centres, notably Belfast (Adams, 1971) and Glasgow (Isaacs, 1977), but doubt exists as to the effectiveness of these stroke units because of a lack of scientific evaluation.

In a comparison of the groups of patients treated 'before' and 'after' a stroke rehabilitation unit had been opened, Hurwitz and Adams (1972) found that a higher proportion of patients treated in the unit could be discharged to community care, with a consequent reduction in the proportion requiring long-term hospital care. Isaacs and Marks (1973) in an account of the work of a stroke rehabilitation unit, concluded that severely disabled stroke patients can respond to prolonged rehabilitation in a suitably organised unit. On the other hand, Waylonis and his colleagues (1973) found that a stroke rehabilitation team introduced into a small community hospital did not have any effect on the functional outcome of patients.

Feldman et al (1972), in a controlled study of the rehabilitation of an unselected group of stroke patients, concluded that there was no advantage in a formal rehabilitation programme, prescribed and managed by a department of physical medicine, compared with 'functionally orientated' medical care. A randomised controlled trial, conducted as part of the Birmingham Stroke Study, compared standard University Hospital care with intensive multidisciplinary rehabilitation (Peacock et al, 1972). The results of intensive rehabilitation were encouraging, but lengthy and expensive rehabilitation did not prove to be of value. The question of what is the most effective method of organising resources for stroke rehabilitation requires to be answered with urgency in view of the growth of the problem.

THE THERAPIST'S APPROACH TO STROKE REHABILITATION

Whatever the arguments for or against stroke units, it seems clear that a multidisciplinary team is required for the treatment of stroke, consisting of physiotherapist, occupational therapist, speech therapist, nurse, social worker and doctor (McLeod and Williamson, 1967; Steinman, 1976). Although group therapy has a place (Redinger et al, 1971; Bullock and Lupton, 1974), stroke victims need individual rehabilitation (Adams, 1974). There is some doubt about what should be the basic approach of the physiotherapist to the individual patient. Various approaches to treatment have been advocated in the past 20 years. Brunnstrom's (1964) treatment is based on the principle that voluntary movement develops as a product of more primitive reflexes, modified in a particular sequence. Once the tonic reflexes integrated in the brain stem are well established, they can be modified and voluntarily inhibited by the patient. Progression of integration to the mid-brain inhibits the tonic response, in favour of the righting reflex. Finally, voluntary movement, integrated at the cortical level, results from this progression. The Bobath (1970) approach also aims for higher cortical control; but whereas Brunnstrom makes use of the abnormal (especially tonic reflexes) through conditioning and modification to permit functional activities, Bobath aims to inhibit the abnormal and facilitate the normal. This is achieved by using 'reflex-inhibiting postures' to change the abnormal patterns of movement produced by abnormal tone, which have to be suppressed before normal ones can be introduced. Reflex-inhibiting movement patterns inhibit abnormal postural reactions and facilitate active automatic and voluntary movements. By controlling part of the abnormal patterns at their most important points only, spasticity can be reduced throughout the body. The Bobath approach emphasises that it is essential to assess the patient's individual problems when planning therapy. Another approach advocated in stroke therapy is proprioceptive neuromuscular facilitation (PNF), first described by Knott (1956). Neurophysiological principles concerned with proprioceptors and the spinal connections, and the supraspinal influences upon the synapse of the anterior horn cells provide the basis for procedures used to activate responses in patients with hemiplegia. The application of these techniques is considered in detail by Manning (1974).

Community health team

The community health care team headed by the general practitioner offers an alternative to hospital treatment only for the mildest strokes. Rehabilitation of stroke patients in their own homes has been successfully attempted in selected patients (Rogoff et al, 1963), but in almost every case the stroke occurred several weeks before admission to the study, by which time the relatives had adjusted to it and were prepared to continue their support. The relatives of over one-third of suitable patients refused to participate in a home-cared programme in spite of the financial advantages which then resulted in the United States from staying out of hospital. The investigation was uncontrolled, and the patients were compared with themselves before and after treatment, so that no conclusions can be drawn as to how well domiciliary rehabilitation of stroke patients compared with treatment in hospital.

EVALUATION OF STROKE REHABILITATION

The problems associated with the evaluation of stroke rehabilitation have been reviewed elsewhere (Garraway, 1976). The following questions will be asked:

WHERE should stroke rehabilitation resources be located?
WHAT is the optimum level of resources that should be deployed?
HOW should stroke rehabilitation be conducted?
WHICH stroke patients will derive the most benefit from rehabilitation?

WHERE should stroke rehabilitation resources be located?
An answer to this question is currently being sought in Edinburgh. A randomised controlled trial has been under way since 1974 in which patients with acute strokes aged 65 years and over are randomly allocated to a stroke rehabilitation unit in a geriatric assessment ward or to one of a number of general medical units. The stroke unit has been set up along the lines of that established at Lightburn Hospital, Glasgow (Isaacs, 1977). This study, the methodology of which has been reported (Garraway et al, 1977), will be completed in 1979. An 'Activities of Daily Living Unit' which can replicate patients' home circumstances has been constructed to provide objective assessment (Smith et al, 1977). The Edinburgh Stroke Study will not provide a definitive measure of the optimum level of manpower or facilities for effective rehabilitation, but will determine whether care in one stroke unit is more successful than care in general medical units.

WHAT is the optimum level of resources for stroke rehabilitation?
Although the benefit of early rehabilitation following stroke is generally accepted (Truscott et al, 1974) there is little evidence to determine what levels of therapy should be prescribed. The level of physiotherapy and speech therapy should almost certainly exceed the 30 min and 10 min per day respectively which Langton Hewer (1972) found were received by acute stroke patients in one hospital. But it is not known at what point the level of input of therapy stops improving the stroke patient's performance. A study which will go some way towards answering this question is being conducted at Northwick Park Hospital (Smith and Meade, 1977). This study, which began in 1972, is a randomised controlled trial of different levels of outpatient treatment following stroke with loss of limb and/or speech function. The Northwick Park Study is using methods of assessing functional ability similar to those used in the Edinburgh ADL Assessment Unit (Benjamin, 1976).

HOW should stroke rehabilitation be conducted?
The evidence of the effectiveness of therapy put forward so far has been based on personal experience, not on scientific evaluation. A survey of 45 hospitals revealed that PNF was used 'often or intensively' in 22 departments and 'rarely' in six; the Bobath approach was used 'often or intensively' in 13 departments but 'rarely or never' in 16 (Hurd, 1975). Multicentre studies are urgently required to answer the claims of the various schools.

WHICH stroke patients derive most benefit from rehabilitation?
A more accurate assessment of functional prognosis following stroke is essential if rehabilitation resources are to be deployed in a more effective manner. This aspect of the natural history of the disease has been studied retrospectively in large, carefully documented series (Marquardsen, 1969; Hurtwitz and Adams, 1972; Lehmann, 1975). Broad conclusions can be drawn from these studies with respect to adverse factors in functional prognosis, but they cannot be used to predict the degree of recovery after stroke with any accuracy. A more hopeful approach is to follow up a cohort of stroke patients prospectively. There are two essential prerequisites for this to be undertaken successfully on a large

multicentre scale. First, there must be agreed criteria of outcome (probably based on ADL indices) which are comprehensive, simple, flexible, objective and reliable (Nichols, 1976). Secondly, a standard form of neurological examination must be adopted, preferably based on a series of simple quantitative scales. This approach has already been shown to be of value in predicting the prognosis during the acute phase following stroke (Tuthill et al, 1969).

Several studies have described results on small series of patients using this approach. Stern and his colleagues (1971) emphasised the poor functional outcome in patients with hemisensory losses in addition to hemiplegia. Newman (1972), using a standard neurological scoring system, described the wide variation of time in which recovery takes place following an acute stroke. Fugl-Meyer and his colleagues (1975) applied a detailed method of assessing motor function to 28 hemiplegic stroke patients, and showed that the return of motor function followed a predictable course. Much work remains to be done in this area before a practical, universally acceptable, standard examination for assessing functional prognosis in stroke emerges. An indication of the problems of observer variability in applying such an examination has recently been given (Garraway et al, 1976). But persistence in developing a suitable neurological examination probably represents the most promising avenue for improving the effectiveness of stroke rehabilitation in the near future.

REFERENCES

Adams, G. F. (1971) Clinical outlook for stroke patients. *Gerontologia clinica*, **13**, 181–188.

Adams, G. F. (1974) *Cerebrovascular Disability and the Ageing Brain*. Edinburgh: Churchill Livingstone.

Adams, G. F. & Hurwitz, L. J. (1963) Mental barriers to recovery after strokes. *Lancet*, **ii**, 533–537.

Allison, R. S. (1962) *The Senile Brain*. London: E. Arnold Ltd.

Anderson, W. F. (1966) The principles and practice of rehabilitation in hemiplegia. *Physiotherapy*, **1**, 34–39.

Benjamin, J. (1976) *Journal of Occupational Therapy*, **39**, 301–306.

Ben-Yishay, Y., Diller, L., Gerstman, L. & Hass, A. (1968) The relationship between impersistence, intellectual function and outcome of rehabilitation in patients with left hemiplegia. *Neurology*, **18**, 852–861.

Bobath, B. (1970) *Adult Hemiplegia: Evaluation and Treatment*. London: Heinemann Medical Books Ltd.

Brocklehurst, J. (1973) *Textbook of Geriatric Medicine and Gerontology*. Edinburgh: Churchill Livingstone.

Brunnstrom, S. (1964) *Movement Therapy in Hemiplegia, a Neurophysiological Approach*. New York: Harper and Row.

Buskirk, C. V. (1954) Return of motor function in hemiplegia. *Neurology*, **4**, 919–928.

Council Working Party (1974) Comments on report of remedial professions. *British Journal of Occupational Therapy*, **37**, 117–119.

Critchley, M. (1955) Personification of paralysed limbs in hemiplegics. *British Medical Journal*, **iii**, 284–287.

Drake, W. E., Hamilton, M. J., Carlsson, M. & Brumenkrantz, J. (1973) Acute stroke management and patient outcome: the value of neurovascular care units. *Stroke*, **4**, 933–945.

Eisenberg, H., Morrison, J. T., Sullivan, E. & Foote, F. M. (1964) Cerebrovascular accidents. Incident and survival rates in a defined population, Middlesex County, Connecticut. *Journal of the American Medical Association*, **189**, 883–888.

Feldman, D. J., Lee, B. R., Untereker, J., Lloyd, K., Rusk, H. A. & Toole, A. (1972) A comparison of functionally orientated medical care and formal rehabilitation in the management of patients with hemiplegia due to cerebrovascular disease. *Journal of Chronic Diseases*, **15**, 297–310.

Ford, J. (1971) Occupational therapy with stroke patients. *Modern Geriatrics*, **1**, 414–422.

Fugl-Meyer, A. R., Jaasko, L., Leyman, I., Olsson, S. & Steglind, S. (1975) The post-stroke patient. 1. A method for evaluation of physical performance. *Scandinavian Journal of Rehabilitation Medicine*, **7**, 13–31.

Garraway, W. M. (1977) Edinburgh Stroke Rehabilitation Study: background and methodology (in preparation).

Garraway, W. M. (1976) Evaluation in the National Health Service. *Health Bulletin*, **34**, 256–261.

Garraway, W. M., Akhtar, A. J., Gore, S. M., Prescott, J. R. & Smith, R. G. (1976) Observer variation in the clinical assessment of stroke. *Age and Ageing*, **5**, 233–240.

Geltner, L. (1972) Comprehensive care of cerebrovascular accidents. *Gerontologia clinica*, **14**, 346–353.

Gersten, J. W. (1967) Evaluation of rehabilitation potential in stroke patients. *Stroke Rehabilitation—Basic Concepts and Research Trends*, ed. Fields, W. S. & Spencer, L. A. St Louis: Warren H. Green.

Gersten, J. W. (1975) *Stroke and its Rehabilitation*, ed. Licht, S. Baltimore: Waverley Press.

Gregory, M. E. & Aitken, M. B. (1971) Assessment of parietal lobe function in hemiplegia. *British Journal of Occupational Therapy*, **34**, 9–16.

Gresham, G. E., Fitzpatrick, T. E., Wolf, P. A., McNamara, P. M., Kannel, W. B. & Dawber, T. R. (1975) Residual disability in survivors of stroke—The Framingham Study. *New England Journal of Medicine*, **293**, 954–956.

Harris, A. I. (1971) *Handicapped and Impaired in Great Britain*. Part 1. Social Survey Division, Office of Population, Censuses and Surveys. London: HMSO.

Hass, A., Rusk, A. H., Pelosof, H. & Adam, R. J. (1967) Respiratory function in hemiplegic patients. *Archives of Physical Medicine and Rehabilitation*, **48**, 174–179.

Heasman, M. A. & Lipworth, L. (1966) *Accuracy of Certification of Cause of Death*. General Registry Office, Studies on Medical and Population Subjects No. 20. London: HMSO.

Hodkinson, H. N. (1972) Evaluation of a mental test score for assessment of mental impairment in the elderly. *Age and Ageing*, **1**, 233–238.

Hurd, S. (1975) Survey of occupational therapy for the hemiplegic patient: trends in treatment methods and media. *Occupational Therapy*, **38**, 81–83.

Hurwitz, L. F. & Adams, G. F. (1972) Rehabilitation of hemiplegia—indices of assessment and prognosis. *British Medical Journal*, **i**, 94–98.

Isaacs, B. (1971) Identification of disability in the stroke patient. *Modern Geriatrics*, **1**, 390–402.

Isaacs, B. (1963) The diagnostic value of tests with toys in old people. *Gerontologia clinica*, **5**, 8–22.

Isaacs, B. & Akhtar, A. J. (1972) The set test—a rapid test of mental function in old people. *Age and Ageing*, **1**, 222–226.

Isaacs, B. & Marks, R. (1973) Determinants of outcome of stroke rehabilitation. *Age and Ageing*, **2**, 139–149.

Isaacs, B. (1973) In *Textbook of Geriatric Medicine and Gerontology* ed. Brocklehurst, J. Edinburgh: Churchill Livingstone.

Isaacs, B. (1977) Five years' experience of a stroke unit. *Health Bulletin*, **35**, 94–98.

Isaacs, B. & Walkey, F. (1963) The assessment of the mental state of elderly hospital patients using a simple questionnaire. *American Journal of Psychiatry*, **120**, 173–174.

Kannel, W. B., Dawber, D. R., Cohen, M. E. & Macnamara, B. N. (1965) Vascular disease of the brain—epidemiologic aspects; the Framingham Study. *American Journal of Public Health*, **55**, 1355–1366.

Katz, S., Ford, B. A., Moskowitz, W. R., Jackson, A. B. & Jaffe, W. M. (1963) Studies of illness in the aged. *Journal of the American Medical Association*, **185**, 914–919.

Kennedy, F. B., Pozen, T. J., Gabelman, E. H., Tuthill, J. E. & Zaentz, S. D. (1970) Stroke intensive care—an appraisal. *American Heart Journal*, **80**, 188–196.

Knott, M. (1967) Introduction to and philosophy of neuromuscular facilitation. *Physiotherapy*, **53**, 2–12.

Kurtzke, J. F. (1969) *Epidemiology of Cerebrovascular Disease*. Berlin: Springer-Verlag.

Hewer, R. L. (1976) In *Stroke. Proceedings of the Ninth Pfizer International Symposium*, ed. Gillingham, F. J., Mawdsley, C. & Williams, A. E. Edinburgh: Churchill Livingstone.

Hewer, R. L. (1973) The management of hemiplegia. *Proceedings of the Royal Society of Medicine*, **66**, 882–884.

Lehmann, J. F., Delateur, B. J., Fowler, R. S., Warren, C. G., Arnhold, R., Schertzer, G., Hurka, R., Whitmore, J. J., Masock, A. J. & Chambers, K. H. (1975) Stroke—does rehabilitation affect outcome? *Archives of Physical Medicine and Rehabilitation*, **56**, 375–382.

Lehmann, J. F., Delateur, B. J., Fowler, R. S., Warren, C. G., Arnhold, R., Scherezer, G., Hurka, R., Whitmore, J. J., Masock, A. J. & Chambers, K. H. (1975) Stroke rehabilitation: outcome and prediction. *Archives of Physical Medicine and Rehabilitation*, **56**, 383–389.

Licht, S. (1975) In *Stroke and its Rehabilitation*, ed. Licht, S. Baltimore: Waverley Press.

Lowman, E. W. (1948) Rehabilitation of the hemiplegic patient. *Journal of the American Medical Association*, **137**, 431–436.

Manning, J. (1974) In *Neurology for Physiotherapists*, ed. Cash, J. London: Faber and Faber.

Marquardsen, J. (1969) *The Natural History of Acute Cerebrovascular Disease*. Copenhagen: Munksgaard.

Martin, J. P. (1967) *The Basal Ganglia and Posture*. London: Pitman.

Matsumoto, N., Whisnant, J. P., Kurland, L. T. & Okazaki, H. (1973) Natural history of stroke in Rochester, Minnesota, 1955 through 1969: an extension of a previous study, 1945 through 1954. *Stroke*, **4**, 20–29.

McLeod, R. D. M. & Williamson, J. (1967) Problems of stroke assessment and rehabilitation. *Scottish Medical Journal*, **12**, 384–405.

Milne, J. S., Maule, M. M., Cormack, S. & Williamson, J. (1972) The design and testing of questionnaire and examination to assess physical and mental health in older people using a staff nurse as the observer. *Journal of Chronic Diseases*, **25**, 385–405.

National Institute of Neurological Diseases and Blindness. Report of an Ad Hoc Committee of the Advisory Council for the US Public Health Service (1958). A classification and outline of cerebrovascular disease. *Neurology (Minneapolis)*, **8**, 395–434.

Newman, M. (1972) The process of recovery after hemiplegia. *Stroke*, **3**, 702–710.

Nichols, P. J. R. (1976) Are ADL indices of any value? *Occupational Therapy*, **39**, 160–163.

Nichols, P. J. R. (1976) *Rehabilitation Medicine*. Butterworth: London.

Overs, B. R. & Belknap, E. L. (1966) Educating stroke patients' families. *Journal of Chronic Disease*, **20**, 45–51.

Patterson, A. (1971) The speech therapist's role in stroke rehabilitation. *Modern Geriatrics*, **1**, 403–407.

Peacock, R. B., Riley, C. P., Lampton, T. D., Raffel, S. S. & Walker, J. S. (1972) The Birmingham Stroke Epidemiology and Rehabilitation Study. In *Trends in Epidemiology*, ed. Stewart, G. T. Springfield: Thomas.

Peszczynski, M. (1961) Prognosis for rehabilitation of the older adult and the aged hemiplegic patient. *American Journal of Cardiology*, **7**, 365–369.

Rankin, J. (1957) Cerebral vascular accidents in patients over the age of 60. II. Prognosis. *Scottish Medical Journal*, **2**, 200–215.

Redinger, R. A., Forster, S., Dolphin, M. K., Godduhn, J. & Weisinger, J. (1971) Group therapy in the rehabilitation of the severely aphasic and hemiplegic in the late stages. *Scandinavian Journal of Rehabilitation Medicine*, **3**, 89–91.

Registrar General for Scotland (1976) *Annual Report 1975. Part 1. Mortality Statistics*. Edinburgh: HMSO.

Rogoff, D. J., Cooney, V. D. & Kutner, B. (1964) Hemiplegia—a study of home rehabilitation. *Journal of Chronic Diseases*, **17**, 539–550.

Royal College of Physicians of London (1974) *Report on Geriatrics Committee Working Group on Strokes*. London: Royal College of Physicians.

Scottish In-Patient Statistics (1975) Information Services Division of the Common Services Agency. Edinburgh: Scottish Health Service.

Sharland, D. E. (1964) Ability of men to return to work after cardiac infarction. *British Medical Journal*, **ii**, 718–720.

Silver, C. B. (1972) Simple methods of testing ability in geriatric patients. *Gerontologia clinica*, **2**, 110–122.

Smith, M. E., Garraway, W. M., Akhtar, A. J. & Andrews, C. J. A. (1977) An assessment unit for measuring the outcome of stroke rehabilitation. *British Journal of Occupational Therapy*, **39**, 51–53.

Smith, D. S. & Meade, T. W. (1977) Personal communication.

Steinmann, B. (1976) Care, rehabilitation and follow-up of the stroke patient. *Age and Ageing*, Supplementary Issue, 31–40.

Stern, P. H., McDowell, F., Miller, J. M. & Robinson, M. (1971) Factors influencing stroke rehabilitation. *Stroke*, **2**, 213–218.

Truscott, B. L., Kretschmann, C. M., Toole, J. F. & Pajak, T. F. (1974) Early rehabilitative care in community hospitals: effect on quality of survivorship following a stroke. *Stroke*, **5**, 623–629.

Tuthill, J. E., Pozen, T. J. & Kennedy, F. B. (1969) A neurologic grading system for acute strokes. *American Heart Journal*, **78**, 53–57.

Twitchell, T. E. (1951) Restoration of motor function in hemiplegia in man. *Brain*, **74**, 443–480.

Ullman, M. (1962) *Behavioural Changes in Patients Following Hemiplegia*. Springfield, Illinois: Thomas.

Veterans Administration Study Group on Antihypertensive Agents (1970) Effects of treatment on morbidity in hypertension: results in patients with diastolic blood pressure averaging 115 through 129 mmHg. *Journal of the American Medical Association*, **202**, 1028–1034.

Veterans Administrative Cooperative Study Group on Antihypertensive Agents (1970) Effects of treatment on morbidity in hypertension: II Results in patients with diastolic pressures averaging 90 through 114 mmHg. *Journal of the American Medical Association*, **213**, 1143–1152.

Waylonis, G. W., Keitu, M. W. & Aseff, J. N. (1973) Stroke rehabilitation in a midwestern county. *Archives of Physical Medicine and Rehabilitation*, **54**, 151–155.

Whisnant, J. P., Fitzgibbon, J. P., Kurland, K. T. & Sayre, G. P. (1971) Natural history of stroke in Rochester, Minnesota, 1945 through 1954. *Stroke*, **2**, 11–22.

Wilson, J. & Agate, J. (1971) Occupational therapy with stroke patients. *Modern Geriatrics*, **1**, 408–413.

World Health Organisation (1969) *Technical Report Series, No. 419*. WHO Export Committee on Medical Rehabilitation. Second Report. Geneva.

World Health Organisation (1971a) Cerebrovascular diseases: prevention, treatment and rehabilitation. *Technical Report Series No. 469*.

World Health Organisation (1975) *World Health Statistics Annual, 1972. Part 1. Vital Statistics and Causes of Death.*

Wylie, M. C. (1960) Delay in seeking rehabilitation after cerebrovascular accident. *Journal of Chronic Diseases*, **13**, 442–451.

Wylie, M. C. (1964) Participation of general practitioners in a rehabilitation program. *Journal of Chronic Diseases*, **17**, 359–369.

2. The investigation and management of incontinence

John Charles Brocklehurst

The urinary bladder might seem to be a relatively simple organ peripherally placed within the body and serving only to contain a moderate quantity of urine and to allow this to be passed without difficulty when time and place are appropriate. Its accessibility to visual and dynamic study and its uniform presence throughout the mammalian world might also suggest that its structure and method of functioning could be easily explored and would by now be well understood. However this is far from being the case, as any acquaintanceship with the vast literature about the urinary bladder will readily confirm. Therefore, before proceeding to consider the specific problem of urinary incontinence in old age, it is necessary to consider current concepts in bladder anatomy and physiology.

PROPERTIES OF THE BLADDER

The urinary bladder normally accommodates about 600 ml of urine and is capable of emptying itself completely. Indeed the completeness of emptying is one of the safeguards against the multiplication of pathogenic organisms within it. It is capable of containing 2 litres and more, but over-distension to that extent will normally be exquisitely painful unless such capacity is reached gradually over a prolonged period of time. In the elderly, however, such over-distension is not always painful.

As the bladder fills up, its muscular wall accommodates to the increase in volume without any significant rise in intravesical pressure. Indeed, when the bladder is filled with 500 ml of urine the true intravesical pressure is likely to be somewhere around 7 to 10 cm of water. There is, of course, the additional element of pressure which will be registered in the bladder but which is transmitted directly from the body cavity. This will be affected by posture and movement—for instance by different phases of respiration, by coughing and by the Valsalva manoeuvre.

As the normal bladder fills up an awareness of distension reaches consciousness at some point beyond 250 ml. Normally no intrinsic contractions of the bladder occur unless they are consciously allowed by the individual in order voluntarily to empty his bladder. How such contractions are prevented and how, indeed, when they occur, the various muscular elements of the bladder and urethra work together to allow its complete emptying, are among those aspects of physiology and anatomy which are still disputed.

In addition the bladder must have a surface which is waterproof and impervious to electrolytes and other substances contained in the urine. The transitional epithelial cells which line the bladder must therefore be able to fold in on themselves when emptying and also become a luminal membrane which remains waterproof when stretched.

The bladder outlet must also be able to remain closed when very high levels of intravesical pressure are transmitted from the body cavity as during coughing, straining, etc.

ANATOMY AND PHYSIOLOGY

Anatomical study of the bladder muscle using conventional techniques continues to be made. The whole subject has been reviewed and brought together by Hutch (1972) in his monograph, *Anatomy and Physiology of the Bladder, Trigone and Urethra.* Hutch reanalyses a number of classical dissections of the bladder and describes a number of dissections of his own. He relates these to x-ray studies (cysto-urethrograms) in developing his theory of the function of the different muscular elements of the bladder. He thus reviews bladder function and also the place of micturating cysto-urethrography as an investigation.

The base plate

Hutch's major contribution has been in defining the 'base plate' which has a sphincteric effect when it is flat and unbroken, but contributes to bladder emptying when it has been broken (see Fig. 2.1). The base plate consists of two elements. The first is the trigone, a triangular extension of the muscle fibres from the ureters which pass down on the surface

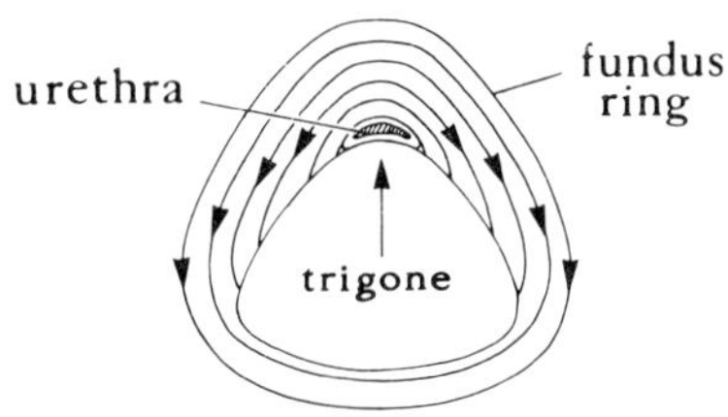

Fig. 2.1 The base plate of the bladder (after Hutch, 1972)

of the detrusor muscles to the lower end of the urethra in the female and the veromontanum in the male. The fibres join together between the ureteric orifices to form the *crista urethralis* (or Mercier's bar). The trigone is mesenchymal in derivation, whereas the remainder of the bladder muscle is endodermal. The second element of the base plate consists of the middle circular fibres of the detrusor, where muscle fibres are so disposed as to maintain the internal urethral orifice closed. Hutch calls this the *fundus ring.* The base plate may be seen on lateral cystograms lying above and parallel to the SCIPP line (the line between the sacro-coccygeal joint and the inferior pubic point). Examination of this area is facilitated by using micturating cysto-urethrography as an investigation of incontinence (see page 26).

The detrusor

The base plate is normally broken by the action upon it of the outer longitudinal fibres of the detrusor muscle (Fig. 2.2). These form two outer principal loops, one anterior and one posterior. Both are inserted into the transverse precervical arc which is described as 'a tough musculofibrous point of insertion' for these two loops which surrounds the anterior one-third of the bladder neck. The anterior longitudinal muscle passes up the ventral surface of the bladder and loops around the urachus. The posterior longitudinal layer of the detrusor consists of a medial and two lateral elements. The two lateral elements originate near the urachus and pass dorsally downward, joining together in front of the bladder outlet to form the detrusor loop. This fuses with the posterior surface of the transverse pre-cervical arc.

The medial part of the posterior outer longitudinal muscle runs from the urachus behind the trigone and inserts into the apex of the deep trigone.

Bladder emptying

Hutch's theory of bladder emptying will now be evident from a consideration of these different muscular elements. Contraction of the medial posterior part of the outer longitudinal muscle will pull the apex of the trigone dorsally and will thus break the base plate. Once the base plate is broken the effect of the fundus ring will be to bring together the lower part of the bladder as a cone of diminishing size. At the same time the anterior and the lateral posterior elements of the outer longitudinal layer of the detrusor, being inserted together into the immovable precervical arc, will, by their contractions in opposing directions, squeeze the dome of the bladder, completing the process of bladder emptying.

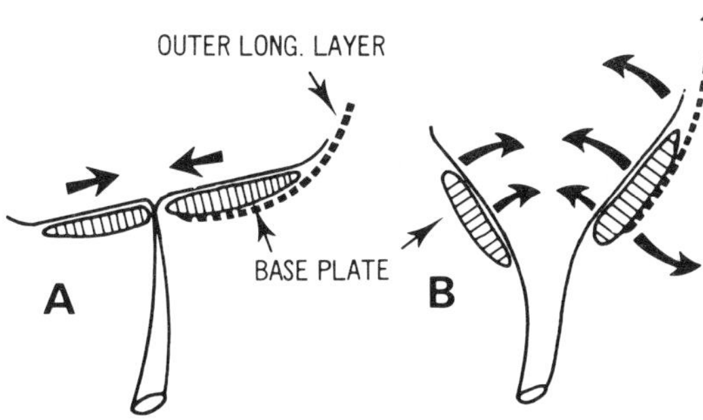

Fig. 2.2 The base plate after it has been broken by contraction of the medial posterior layer of the outer longitudinal detrusor muscle (after Hutch, 1972)

The trigone

The trigone itself consists of superficial and deep layers and it is the deep layer which continues into the posterior wall of the urethra. According to Hutch the deep trigone also forms part of the anterior urethral tissue in the lower part of the female urethra and at the level of the veromontanum in the male. Wessen's (1920) concept of bladder muscle function which is supported by Tanagho, Smith and Meyers (1968) and by Woodburne (1968) is that the trigone is involved in the initiation of micturition, a function which is easily understood from its morphology. This, in terms of Hutch's theory, would contribute towards the breaking of the base plate. Others, however, believe that the trigone functions only to prevent retrograde ejaculation in the male.

Autonomic nerves

A more recent approach to bladder anatomy has been based on deductions made from neurohistochemical techniques associated with electron microscopy by Gosling and Dixon (1975). These studies led them to the hypothesis that there are distinct structural differences between the detrusor smooth muscle and the muscle surrounding the bladder neck and proximal urethra. They found cholinesterase positive (presumptive cholinergic) nerve endings in both areas; whereas noradrenergic nerve endings were detected only in the neck and urethra but not in the fundus and body of the bladder. By electron microscopy they demonstrated smooth muscle cells in large bundles, separated from each other by numerous collagen fibres in the fundus, but occurring singly or in small groups in the bladder neck and proximal urethra. They suggested that detrusor contractions can occur without directly inducing contraction of the smooth muscle of the bladder neck and proximal urethra, and vice versa. They thus incline to the classical theory of reciprocal sympathetic/parasympathetic innervation of the bladder and its sphincter, which has been out of fashion for the last 30 years.

Additional evidence for the function of the sympathetic nervous system in contributing towards the closure of the urethra and the maintenance of continence has been brought by Rohner et al (1971) and Nergardh (1975). Pharmacological experiments have shown that alpha-adrenergic blockade by phentolamine leads to a drop in urethral pressure (Whitfield et al, 1976; Andersen and Bradley, 1976b). It is possible that this is due to diminishing vascularity of the tissues surrounding the urethra (Tulloch, 1974). Beta-adrenergic innervation does not seem to be involved in bladder function (Whitfield et al, 1976; Benson et al, 1976). There still seems to be no doubt that the main element in contraction of the bladder fundus is cholinergic, as shown by pelvic nerve stimulation (Diokno, Davies and Lapides, 1973).

Mechanical effect of tissues

In addition to the purely muscular effect in maintaining the closure of the bladder outlet it is clear that the tissues surrounding the urethra contain a large amount of collagen (elastic fibres) as well as a considerable vascular element. Woodburne (1968) has suggested that the elastic and mechanical properties contribute about 40 per cent and Downey and Awad (1976) that they contribute 60 per cent to the forces maintaining closure of the urethra.

The striated muscle

The striated muscle of the pelvic diaphragm and the external sphincter do not normally contribute to the maintenance of continence. The external sphincter can be extinguished by will, even with a full bladder, and no micturition occurs (Sundin and Peterson, 1975). Indeed it has been known for many years that the external sphincter may be removed or its pudenal nerve supply abolished without impairing continence (Langworthy, Kolb and Lewis, 1940; Emmett, Dant and Dunn, 1948; Ardran et al 1967). Recent electromyographic studies of the urogenital diaphragm have shown that in the resting stage it maintains complete electrical silence, or else there is slow discharge of one or two motor units only. Activity increases during bladder filling and reaches its maximum when the bladder is full (Diokno, Coff and Bender, 1974). The striated muscle element in the bladder outlet is occasionally a problem when there is incoordination between its relaxation and the contracting emptying bladder (see below).

The smooth muscle

There is very little information as to the effect of ageing on the smooth muscle cells of the bladder itself. Brent and Stephens (1975) showed that in the rabbit these muscle cells may increase not only in size but also in number as a reaction to obstruction. This suggests that they are not fixed postmitotic cells as has usually been thought. It is possible that the main contribution to age change in the bladder wall itself is in the connective tissue element, and that the well-known changes with cross-linking in elastic fibres contribute to impaired bladder function as well as affecting the periurethral tissue. However, no research has been reported on ageing in these situations.

The epithelium

Apart from studies related to the function of transitional epithelium (Cooper, 1972; Hicks, 1975) the principal interest in the epithelium of the bladder has centred on the development of oestrogen-sensitive stratified squamous epithelium in the urethra and trigone. Reports of the increasing formation of stratified squamous epithelium in these situations have been available for many years (Zuckerman, 1940; Tyler, 1962; Packham, 1971). More recent contributions have described these in greater detail. Henry and Fox (1971) describe a greyish, heaped-up mucosa with a serpiginous margin surrounded by a cuff of hyperaemia occurring in the trigone of women aged 15 to 73. This epithelium, being the result of non-keratinising squamous metaplasia, contained vacuoles and glycogen, showed sudden change to transitional epithelium at its edge, and was oestrogen-sensitive. It has been described as pseudomembranous trigonitis, which may occur in the absence of infection (Streitz, 1963). It is not yet entirely clear whether the disposition of this oestrogen-sensitive epithelium is related to the embryological origins of the urethra and trigone from the mesodermal Woolfian system, or to the effect of ectodermal elements (Bulmer, 1959).

The effect of ageing on oestrogen-sensitive stratified squamous epithelium has been described from studies of vaginal cytology by Meisels (1966). Stoll (1954) shows the variation which is found postmenopausally. Forty-nine per cent of his patients showed androgenic type of change, 37 per cent atrophic change and 14 per cent oestrogenic. That this affects the urethra as well as the genital areas has been shown by Smith (1972), Von Rutte and Delinon (1968), Smith, Roberts and Slade (1970) and Youngblood et al (1958).

DIAGNOSTIC METHODS

The last 10 years have seen enormous strides in the development of methods to record bladder pressure and flow. A large number of centres in the UK are now equipped to undertake urodynamic studies on incontinent patients.

The cystometrogram

The cystometrogram has been known and used for 100 years, but now for the first time it is possible to measure simultaneously the intravesical and intra-abdominal pressure (measured as the rectal pressure) and to record the pressure which remains when the intra-abdominal pressure is subtracted from the intravesical pressure. This is the *subtracted bladder pressure* and is a true recording of the pressure within the bladder and its variation with intrinsic bladder contractions. It excludes all pressure changes which take place as a result of movements, changes in posture, coughing, etc.

This system has been further developed to provide a simultaneous visual record of these three pressure lines (vesical, rectal and subtracted) together with an indication of the rate and degree of bladder filling and the rate and degree of bladder emptying. All of this is combined on a screen with a simultaneous picture of the bladder itself, obtained by video-cysto-urethrography (Fig. 2.3). Since the whole of this is recorded on videotape it is possible to play it back as many times as is desired to obtain still pictures at any point (Bates, 1971; Bates et al, 1970).

Procedure

The normal procedures for use of this combined cystometry and cysto-urethrography are for the bladder to be filled at variable rates (rapid fill is 100–150 ml/min, a slower fill 50 ml/min) with the patient supine, to register the point at which the patient feels discomfort, to note any uninhibited bladder contractions and, if these occur, to see if the patient is able to inhibit them by voluntary effort. A maximum degree of filling is reached when the patient experiences discomfort or when leakage occurs. The process is then undertaken again, and with the bladder about two-thirds full a number of provocative tests are used (e.g. changing the patient from the lying to the standing position and getting her to cough a number of times) to see whether any of these fires off an intrinsic bladder contraction. Thereafter the patient is asked to pass water, the flow rate is recorded, and the

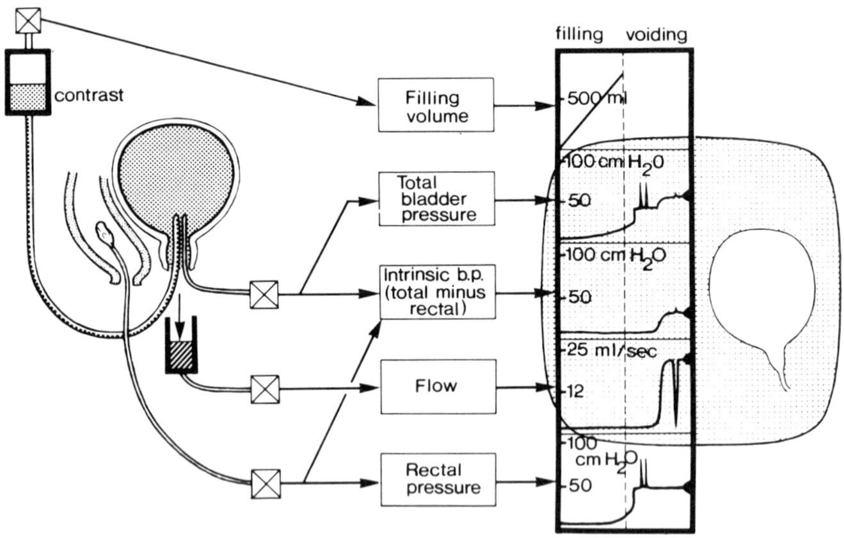

Fig. 2.3 The system used in simultaneous cysto-urethrography, flow measurement and cystography (after Bates, C. P. et al, 1970)

shape of the bladder outlet during micturition is observed. This procedure will identify most types of neurogenic bladder or the unstable bladder (see below) and will also differentiate between genuine stress incontinence and apparent stress incontinence due to an unstable bladder. The flow rate will also suggest whether there is any bladder outlet obstruction.

Normal findings

The whole procedure and normal findings are described by Whiteside and Arnold (1975). Stanton (1972) defines the normal female cystometrogram pattern with filling at 50 ml/min; capacity is 500 ml, desire to void occurs at 150 ml, strong desire to void at 400 ml, maximum voiding pressure is 60 cm of water, and peak flow rate is 30 ml/s.

Gas cystometrography

Further developments have led to the use of a gas-filled system (using carbon dioxide) which allows a filling rate of up to 300 ml/min and 5 to 10 repeat examinations (Bradley et al, 1975, 1976). This is thought to be useful particularly in looking for positional hyperreflexia.

Uro-flow meter

The uro-flow meter may be used apart from the above combined apparatus. Quite often it is not possible to get a patient to pass urine during the somewhat public circumstances of the cystometrogram examination, and the uro-flow meter can then be used in greater privacy (Randall, 1975).

Electromyography

A further development, used more for research than in routine assessment, is the simultaneous recording of the cystometrogram and the electromyograph (Diokno, Koss and Anderson, 1976). This has allowed observations to be made on the part played by the striated muscle during bladder filling and micturition. Attempts have also been made to procure EMG recording of smooth muscles.

Urethral pressure profile

A further investigation which has been developed in the last 10 years is the urethral pressure profile (UPP) (Edwards and Malvern, 1974). This is usually obtained by slowly withdrawing a catheter with a side orifice from the bladder to the vulva, and at the same time bleeding through it sterile water at a slow rate of 2+ ml/min. The urethral pressure profile equipment is also available with a gas-filled system (Andersen and Bradley, 1976a; Tscholl, Tetamanti and Worsdorfer, 1976). The urethral pressure profile is a record of the closing pressure of the urethra, as shown by the resistance offered to the outflow of the small quantity of fluid or gas. The rate of withdrawal of the catheter is noted. Special equipment is now available to remove it at a constant rate (Harrison and Constable, 1970). The UPP also indicates the maximal closing pressure of the urethra, which is generally found at the midpoint, and which is thought to indicate the main disposition of the muscle fibres of the external sphincter. In addition, the UPP shows the pressure throughout the rest of the urethra, and allows a number of measurements to be made for comparison, such as length, maximum closing pressure and the total area of the profile. The reproducibility of UPPs in the same individual has been confirmed by Harrison and Constable (1970). There is still a difference of opinion about the usefulness of this measurement in defining different clinical states. It indicates a shortened urethra in genuine stress incontinence and a low maximal closing pressure in this condition; a high closing pressure in spasticity of the external sphincter and in urethral strictures; and variable changes in other conditions.

Non-invasive methods

All of these are invasive techniques, in as much as they require the passage of a catheter or suprapubic tube into the bladder. Attempts have been made to find a method of measuring residual urine by non-invasive methods. Most commonly used is a method involving I 131 orthoiodohippurate (Strauss and Blaufox, 1970). These workers have confirmed by this method that normally there is no residual urine at all. In 20 patients with various types of obstructive uropathies they found an average residual urine of 77 ml, with a standard deviation of 17 ml. Some estimate of residual urine is also obtainable using the ultrasonogram, and no doubt such a measurement will be obtainable in the future by whole-body scanning.

Future of urodynamic studies

There is an awakening interest among geriatricians, urologists and gynaecologists in urodynamic studies which seems likely to lead in future to a much more precise diagnosis of patients with incontinence (Crisp, Green and Ashken, 1976). This is promoting not only an interest in the subject but also vastly improved management. Unfortunately, there is still a great deal of disagreement as to the part played by different elements of the bladder and the urethra in the process of micturition, and the significance of derangements of this system.

PHARMACOLOGY OF THE BLADDER

The effect of drugs on the bladder has long been of interest in identifying the function of various neurotransmitting agents and in the therapeutic application of such agents and their various antagonists in different types of bladder function disorders. The advent of the alpha- and beta-adrenergic antagonists and stimulators has encouraged further experiments.

Innervation

The fundus or body of the bladder contains both cholinergic and alpha-adrenergic fibres. The bladder base or trigone is poor in cholinergic fibres but has strong alpha-adrenergic representation. Beta-adrenergic fibres play little part in micturition.

Prostaglandins and bromocriptine

Two drugs which have recently been shown to have some possible effect on the bladder and which are presently undergoing further investigation are the prostaglandins (Abrams and Feneley, 1976) and bromocriptine (Farrar and Osborne, 1976). The prostaglandins can be found in seminal vesicle fluid but can also be isolated from many mammalian tissues. They increase bowel motility, initiate and maintain uterine contractions and in the bladder they cause muscle contraction of an order similar to acetyl choline. This effect however is slow and prolonged and probably not a neurotransmitter effect, but something quite different. Bromocriptine (an ergot derivative) has been shown to have some symptomatic effect on the unstable bladder.

Therapeutic applications

Generally the therapeutic application of bladder pharmacology has not changed greatly in the last few years. Anticholinergic drugs have been used for probably a century in the treatment of enuresis—beginning with belladonna, then atropine and subsequently propantheline and emepronium bromide. Emepronium bromide is thought to have a dual effect, blocking transmission both at the peripheral ganglion and at the myoneural junction. Its usefulness in the uninhibited neurogenic bladder and the irritable bladder has been amply confirmed—although a number of workers have reported side-effects, particularly mucosal erosions in the mouth and oesophagus (Brocklehurst et al, 1969; Brocklehurst, Armitage and Jouhar, 1972; Habshaw and Bennett, 1972; Strouthidis, Mankikar and Irvine, 1972). More recently the drug flavoxate, described as having a direct antagonistic effect in the bladder muscle receptor itself, has been used in similar conditions with success and without side-effects (Kohler and Morales, 1968). A double blind crossover trial comparing emepronium bromide and flavoxate in patients with unstable bladders was reported by Stanton (1972), who showed that both were effective in increasing bladder capacity and that flavoxate seemed to be better. Since these two drugs are described as acting at different parts of the autonomic outflow it would seem reasonable to combine them, although no reports of such combinations have yet been made.

The alpha-receptor stimulator, orciprenaline, has also been used in the expectation that it would help to maintain closure of the bladder outlet. Brown et al (1976) compared emepronium, orciprenaline and a combination of these two and showed a rank order as follows in degree of improvement:

Placebo	36 per cent
Orciprenaline	45 per cent
Emepronium	52 per cent
Orciprenaline + emepronium	65 per cent

There were some cardiovascular side-effects with orciprenaline, and gastrointestinal side-effects with emepronium. A cystometrogram study was inconclusive in determining the relative effects of each.

A spastic external sphincter is an occasional problem in incontinence associated with paraplegia (Diokno et al 1976; Sundin and Peterson, 1975). Phenoxibenzamine hydrochloride has been described as being successful in overcoming the problems arising from the spastic external urethral sphincter (Raz and Smith, 1976).

Side-effects on the bladder of other drugs

Intravenous digitalis has been shown to diminish bladder capacity in normal and neurogenic bladders, to provoke a desire to void at a lesser degree of bladder filling and to lead to an increase in intravesical pressure (Sadoughi et al, 1975). It is therefore conceivable that digitalis adds to the bladder problems of some elderly people. Morphine and pethidine have also been shown to increase intravesical pressure, and so has diazepam given by mouth, but not intravenously (Doyle and Biscow, 1976).

THE NEUROGENIC BLADDER

The last 10 years have seen a number of further classifications added to the already complex area of the neurogenic bladder, or neuropathic bladder as it is now being called. To understand the relevance of these different classifications, it is most satisfactory to start from one which is simple and has long been accepted. McLennan in 1939 described the effects on the bladder of the diseases of the central nervous system acting at different levels between the cerebral cortex and the bladder itself. His classification of the neurogenic bladder was as follows:

The autonomous neurogenic bladder

In this case the destruction of the second, third and fourth sacral segments of the spinal cord completely decentralises the bladder, rendering it void of sensation. The bladder partly empties itself from time to time as a result of local contractions leaving a residual urine.

The atonic neurogenic bladder
This type of bladder occurs in disease of the posterior horn cell or the posterior nerve root. Because of loss of sensation the bladder becomes chronically over-distended and atonic. Retention of urine with overflow incontinence results.

The reflex neurogenic bladder
This occurs in a lesion above the sacral segment of the cord but below the bladder centre in the cerebral cortex, most commonly a transection of the spinal cord. The bladder centre in the sacral cord remains intact and so the bladder fills and empties itself reflexly. There is of course no sensation.

The uninhibited neurogenic bladder
In this case the bladder centre in the cingulate gyrus of the frontal cerebral cortex is damaged. Sensation is retained, but the ability is lost to inhibit those bladder contractions which occur as a result of stimulation of the reflex through the sacral centre and which arise as a result of distension. A sensation of impending micturition arises during uninhibited bladder contractions. Since these may continue until they cause emptying, the symptoms of this condition are urgency and urge incontinence.

Types of neurogenic bladder in old age

In old age the uninhibited neurogenic bladder, by far the commonest type, occurs in cerebrovascular disease and senile dementia and possibly as a result of ageing itself. The atonic bladder occurs with peripheral neuropathy, particularly in association with diabetes. The reflex and autonomic neurogenic bladders arise rarely from diseases of the spinal cord such as secondary carcinoma or infarct of the lower end of the cord.

Stable and unstable bladders

An *unstable bladder* is one which shows uninhibited bladder contractions during simple filling or following some provocative stimulus such as a change in intra-abdominal pressure due to coughing, standing or walking. The stable bladder is one in which no intrinsic bladder contraction arises. The unstable bladder includes both the reflex and the uninhibited neurogenic bladder. Intrinsic bladder contractions may also result from purely local causes such as prostatic hypertrophy, the after-effects of gynaecological surgery and possibly infection. The concept of the unstable bladder is useful in differentiating genuine stress incontinence from bladder emptying immediately following coughing or movement (see below).

Another and somewhat similar classification is that of hyperreflexia and areflexia (Bradley et al, 1976) which would seem to offer no advantage over 'stable' and 'unstable'.

Detrusor-sphincter dyssynergia

Detrusor-sphincter dyssynergia occurs in spinal cord disease in association with upper motor neurone lesions (Andersen and Bradley, 1976a). Bladder contractions are associated with clonic contractions of the striated fibres of the external sphincter. This leads to a degree of residual urine and bladder distension. Spasticity of the external sphincter has also been described by Raz and Smith (1976), arising from neurogenic factors, infection, local irritation, diseases of the rectum and pelvic disease.

The bladder in diabetes

The bladder associated with diabetes has been described by Buck et al (1974) in 40 patients, 30 of whom showed cystometrographic changes, related to the severity but not to the duration of diabetes. The changes were those of the atonic bladder with a large capacity and diminished sensation. Total loss of sensation was rare, but consequent infection was common.

Chronic retention of urine

Chronic retention of urine in elderly females has been described by Fox, Jarvis and Henry (1976). The causes included a tight external urethral meatus. Brocklehurst (1977) described a series of aged women with chronic retention associated with the use of anticholinergic drugs, faecal impaction and diabetes.

Bladder outlet obstruction leads to hypertrophy of the muscle bundles of the detrusor, a condition described as trabeculation, which is easily discovered cystoscopically, and on a micturating cystogram. This is followed by the formation of pseudodiverticula and eventually of diverticula. The bladders of elderly women often show diverticula (Parvinen, Sourander and Vuorinen, 1965; Brocklehurst and Dillane, 1967). Brent and Stephens (1975) have shown in rabbits that the smooth muscle cells of the bladder increase in size and number as a reaction to outlet obstruction.

THE DIFFERENTIAL DIAGNOSIS OF URINARY INCONTINENCE IN OLD AGE

A systematic approach to differential diagnosis may best be done by considering disorders at four levels, the pelvic diaphragm, the urethra and bladder outlet, within the bladder itself and in the nervous control of the process of micturition.

Disease of the pelvic diaphragm

In patients with genuine stress incontinence there is weakness of the bladder outlet because of inadequate support from the pelvic floor. The base plate is funnelled rather than flat and there may be effective shortening of the urethra. Radej et al (1976) showed that the functional urethral length (that is urethral length standing minus urethral length lying) was related to the presence of stress incontinence. In 57 patients with stress incontinence the mean functional urethral length was −3.2 mm; whereas in 23 patients with irritable bladder it was +2.7 mm.

When intra-abdominal pressure rises the bladder is squeezed passively. The rise in intravesical pressure which results overcomes the diminished resistance of the bladder outlet and urethra, and a small quantity of urine is lost. It is important to differentiate this condition from the unstable bladder since the treatment is quite different. In many cases the diagnosis can be made by simple inspection of the vulva. A urethral pressure profile of low pressure and short length favours genuine stress incontinence; while the unstable bladder can be diagnosed by cystometrogram.

Disorders of the urethra and bladder outlet

These include stricture, prostatic hypertrophy, the effect of faecal impaction and, in females, abacterial urethritis associated with senile (atrophic) vaginitis. The presence of oestrogen-sensitive epithelium in the urethra has already been discussed; and in states of oestrogen deprivation this may become reddened and granular with associated dysuria (Geist and Salmon, 1943).

Disorders of the bladder itself

These include tumours, calculi and, most commonly, infection. The part which infection of the urine plays in causing incontinence is controversial. Brocklehurst et al (1968) and Milne et al (1972) agree that in total population surveys there is no statistically significant correlation between incontinence and urinary infection. A survey of patients in long-stay geriatric wards showed an association between infection and incontinence (Brocklehurst et al, 1977), but the incontinence was probably the cause of the infection rather than vice versa. There are two reasons for this: first, an association with faecal contamination of the perineum; and secondly, the fact that incontinence due to the uninhibited neurogenic bladder is associated with residual urine which forms a reservoir for the continuation of urinary infection. Similar findings were demonstrated by Macmillan (1972). The importance of residual urine as a cause of infection was discussed by Shand et al (1970), who also draw attention to its increase with age.

Despite this, every practising geriatrician knows that some cases of incontinence are caused simply by the presence of acute urinary infection, and that sterilisation of the urine in these cases eliminates the incontinence. The number of cases of this type is probably quite small, and is not sufficient in epidemiological surveys to show a significant relationship between incontinence and infection.

Disorders of the neurological control of micturition

That the uninhibited neurogenic bladder is the commonest bladder abnormality in incontinence in old age has been demonstrated by several workers (Brocklehurst and Dillane, 1967; Wilson, 1948; Thompson, 1964). Other symptoms of disordered micturition associated with ageing, e.g. nocturnal frequency (Brocklehurst et al, 1968), are due to some degree of uninhibited neurogenic bladder. The evidence is based on the demonstration of cystometrograms characteristic of the uninhibited neurogenic bladder in a series of non-incontinent elderly females (Brocklehurst and Dillane, 1966a), and on the effectiveness of anticholinergic drugs (e.g. emepronium bromide) in diminishing nocturnal frequency (Brocklehurst et al, 1969). In some of these patients there was evidence of upper motor neurone lesions but in others there was no abnormality. It was assumed that in these cases the effect of ageing on cortical neuronal cells, especially in the area of the bladder centre in the cingulate gyrus, diminished the inhibitory effect of this centre. This association of diminished function with increasing age may be compared to other decrements in function which are age-related, such as memory and control of sway. It is assumed therefore that some degree of the uninhibited neurogenic bladder is common as people grow older, and that this accounts for increasing nocturnal frequency and daytime urgency, and predisposes to incontinence when a precipitating factor is added, such as becoming bedfast and dependent on nurses (Brocklehurst, 1951).

This concept still seems the most rational basis for the explanation of incontinence among elderly people, other than those with overt neurological disease. However, the unstable bladder may in some old people be associated not so much with disease of the brain as with local disease (abacterial urethritis, prostatic enlargement and infection).

The importance of the atonic neurogenic bladder as a cause of incontinence has been referred to.

TREATMENT OF INCONTINENCE

Treatment of genuine stress incontinence

Several authors have claimed success with the treatment of stress incontinence by pelvic floor exercises, with or without electronic stimulation. The importance of the pubo-coccygeus muscle in this regard has been stressed by Kegal (1956), who, in 1948, devised a 'perineometer'. This apparatus measures the amount of 'squeeze' which can be applied within the vagina, and thus the effective contraction of the pelvic floor. Pelvic floor exercises have been described by Montgomery (1974) and Harrison (1973). Moore and Schofield (1967) described the use of maximal contraction by faradic stimulation under general anaesthesia, a form of treatment which has not been widely adopted. The use of intermittent faradic stimulation in conscious patients in association with pelvic floor exercises is now generally accepted (Blundell and Smith, 1968; Tanner, 1969).

More recently interferential treatment has been developed. The electronic stimulator in implanted form for anal incontinence was first described by Caldwell (1967), and its use as a pessary by Alexander and Rowan (1968). The whole subject of the electronic control of stress incontinence has been well reviewed by Edwards (1976) and Glen (1975).

If electrical and physiotherapy control of stress incontinence is not successful then gynaecological surgery may be required. A large number of operations have been reviewed by Hodkinson (1965).

Treatment of senile urethritis

Senile urethritis is treated by oestrogens, either by mouth, in the form of ethinyloestradiol tablets or by local application of stilboestrol cream. Local application obviates the clotting risk of oral oestrogen, but is not always easily accomplished in the very old.

Urethral dilation by bougies was described in the treatment of this condition by Roberts and Smith (1968) but is not usually required unless obstruction is apparent during catheterisation.

Treatment of retention

The treatment of chronic retention with bethanecol chloride was described by Lapides (1964). He began with four-hourly subcutaneous injections and gradually changed to oral administration by tablets, with regular measurement of residual urine until the bladder was virtually empty. More recently the drug distigmine bromide (Ubretid) has been used for this purpose and a number of clinical trials from Japan (Condo, 1968; Chiba et al, 1967; Njima and Asano, 1967) show it to be effective in the management of the atonic neurogenic bladder. This drug may also be given intramuscularly (0.5 ml) or by mouth (5 mg daily). Nausea, diarrhoea and blurring of vision have been described.

Urethral dilatation in chronic retention was described by Fox, Jarvis and Henry (1976) in 11 patients with bladder neck stenosis, of whom four were cured and three improved; and by Essenhigh, Ardran and Cope (1968), in 17 women with recurrent cystitis, of whom 10 were improved or relieved of their symptoms. Smith et al (1970) described successful treatment in a large series of patients with urinary symptoms associated with trabeculation and urethral or bladder outlet obstruction.

The use of prolonged bladder distension in the management of patients with unstable bladders has also been described. The bladder is distended by water run into a balloon within the bladder, until a pressure equal to the systolic blood pressure is reached. This pressure is maintained for a period of half an hour. The procedure is repeated on three or four occasions. The rationale is to promote bladder ischaemia, and presumably thereby to diminish the sensitivity of the bladder stretch receptors. Mayo et al (1973) described intracellular collagen following over-distension in experiments with rabbits and in patients who had suffered retention. Mayo and his colleagues (1973) described 12 cases of unstable bladder treated by this method with moderate symptomatic improvement in two, but no change in the cystometrogram. The use of bladder distension was also described by Dunn, Smith and Ardrangn (1974) in 20 cases, of whom 12 were reported as cured and 5 improved; and by Whitfield and Mayo (1975), in 12 patients with no real improvement while rupture of the bladder occurred in one patient. There thus seems to be no case for this form of treatment at present, particularly in view of its risks and its doubtful rationale.

General management of incontinence

The general management of elderly patients with incontinence and the use of pads, appliances and catheters has been surveyed in two publications by the Disabled Living Foundation—*Incontinence* (Mandelstan, 1977) and *The Management of Incontinence in the Home* (Dobson, 1974). Mandelstan's publication is a description of clothing, appliances and pads, whereas Dobson's is a survey of 77 people who were incontinent. Sixty-six of them were referred from local authority welfare departments and 10 replied independently as a result of publicity. Dobson found that many incontinent patients were unwilling to be interviewed and this may be a reflection of the general secrecy and shame surrounding the subject. The people seen were mainly immobile but mentally alert. Cerebrovascular accident and multiple sclerosis were the most common diagnoses. More than half of those interviewed seemed to have had no form of investigation or treatment, receiving such negative comments from their doctors as, 'you have to learn to live with it'. Of the 66 patients, 10 had indwelling catheters and 42 used pads or pants. Many of them were dissatisfied with these. It was noted that patients who used pads had infected urine, together with excoriation of the skin, whereas those who used catheters had infected urine but their skin was not affected. The problems of disposable items and of incontinent laundry facilities were discussed in this report. Laundering is a major problem with uncontrolled incontinence in the home. It is quite clear from this survey that the primary shortcoming in the management of incontinence lies in the education of doctors and nurses. They are ignorant of many of the methods of management and are misinformed about many of those that they use or have heard of.

Catheters

The use of indwelling catheters in intractable urinary incontinence is generally accepted as satisfactory, especially in women, providing thorough examination, diagnosis and specific treatment are first undertaken. The silicone-coated catheter has had a mixed reception. Wastling (1972) documented seven patients who were changed to silicone-coated catheters; all except one had the catheter changed within three weeks because of blockage, one of these within four days. However, the same author, with the experience of a further 18 months (Wastling, 1974) showed that in 15 patients observed over 12 months, the average time between changes of catheter was five months. This evidence clearly shows that the success of silicone-coated catheters depends not so much on the catheter as on the management. Brocklehurst and Brocklehurst (1977) observed 18 elderly long-stay patients for periods of from 8 to 37 weeks. Only one-third of silicone-coated and latex Foley catheters were changed routinely; almost two-thirds were changed because of leakage. Treating the urine with short courses of antibiotics or with six-week courses of the urinary antiseptic, Hiprex, made no difference in the maintenance of sterility of the urine, nor did this diminish the number of occasions on which leakage occurred. However, when weekly bladder washouts were introduced leakage diminished significantly. With a regime of weekly bladder washouts (e.g. with Noxyflex 1 per cent 100 ml) a silicone-coated catheter may be maintained in situ for a long time.

Arising from this the effect of chemical washouts of the bladder has to be considered. Harper and Matz (1975) investigated in the rat the effect of exposure to chlorhexidine solution 1 in 5000 to 1 in 10 000 for 20 to 24 h. Osmotic injury secondary to alteration in the integrity of the lipoprotein membrane was demonstrated. Further studies of this question are needed.

Catheter-induced inflammation in the urethra was studied by Edwards and Trott (1973) who showed that all catheters produced some pus cells in the urethra. Inflammation was greatest during the first two days after catheterisation but diminished the longer the catheter was in situ. There was no relationship between the degree of inflammation and the size or type of catheter. Latex and silicone-coated catheters were compared by Bruce et al (1974). The latter showed very much less encrustation. The amount of encrustation was not related to the length of time the catheter was in use, but individual patients showed marked variation, independent of the type of catheter.

The 'Shepherd sporran' is a collecting bag worn on a belt round the lower part of the body, rather than on the leg. This stays in position much more satisfactorily, and eliminates the occurrences of the filled and heavy bag being suspended from the balloon resting on the bladder base. A bag attached to furniture or lying on the floor is unacceptable in geriatric practice.

Perhaps the most interesting development in long-term catheterisation, but one which is not relevant to the elderly, has been the introduction of self-catheterisation in patients of all ages with atonic bladders (Lapides et al 1974, 1976; Orikasa et al, 1976). These patients keep ordinary catheters in their handbags, unsterilised, and insert them as required, every few hours. The rationale is that infection is not of serious consequence, provided that the bladder is regularly emptied completely. Experience with intermittent self-catheterisation seems to bear this out.

The use of disposable incontinence pads has been well described by Willington (1975, 1976). He estimated that the consumption of incontinence underpads in the United Kingdom was about 120 million a year, at a cost of about £4 million. Generally, they are not satisfactory because they absorb urine but are not able to remove it from contact with the skin. As the patient lies on the pad, urine collects in the depression under the sacrum and buttocks. Most pads are not sealed on all four sides, and therefore the urine seeps or trickles down over the unsealed side and wets the bed. The pad is often unnecessarily large, which serves to spread the wet surface over larger areas of the patient's skin. There are problems of storage and disposal of these large pads.

Willington introduced the marsupial pad which is worn in 'Kanga' pants. These were the subject of a report by the Welsh Hospital Board in 1972 who showed that a year's supply of pads and pants cost at that time £36.34. In a trial of 39 garments among elderly patients in a geriatric unit and mentally defective children, they found complete success in 28 and some leakage in 11. The marsupial pants are made of a knitted hydrophobic material, they do not absorb urine and are not impervious to sweat. They must be very carefully fitted.

The urine is passed into a pad through the hydrophobic material and the pouch in which this pad is carried is waterproof. There seems little doubt that this is the most effective type of pad for general use in urinary incontinence. It is matched only by the gelling pad—incontinence pads containing carboxymethylcellulose (Smith, 1971). These were tested in 27 patients, in half of whom they absorbed the urine satisfactorily for periods of up to 8 h during the day, while 80 per cent of the patients found them suitable for overnight use.

CONCLUSION

Interest in this very important, but much neglected, clinical problem is now increasing. The International Continence Society, with its annual meeting and its lead in standardising nomenclature, is also playing a part. Much new work may be anticipated during the next few years, including further epidemiological studies.

REFERENCES

Abrams, P. H. & Feneley, R. C. L. (1976) The action of prostaglandins on the smooth muscle of the human urinary tract in vitro. *British Journal of Urology*, **47**, 909.

Alexander, S. & Rowan, D. (1968) An electric pessary for stress incontinence. *Lancet*, **ii**, 728.

Andersen, J. T. & Bradley, W. E. (1976a) The syndrome of detrusor sphincter dyssynergia. *Journal of Urology*. **116**, 493.

Andersen, J. T. & Bradley, W. E. (1976b). The urethral pressure profile by a new technique using gas and simultaneous EMG recording. *British Journal of Urology*, **48**, 341.

Ardran, G. M., Cope, V., Essenheigh, D. M. & Tuckey, M. (1967) The primary vesical sphincter. *British Journal of Urology*, **39**, 329.

Bates, C. P. (1971) Continence and incontinence—a clinical study of the dynamics of voiding and of the sphincter mechanism. *Annals of the Royal College of Surgeons of England*, **49**, 18.

Bates, C. P., Whiteside, C. G. & Turner Warwick, R. (1970) Synchronous cine/pressure/flow/cysto-urethrography with special reference to stress in urge incontinence. *British Journal of Urology*, **42**, 714.

Benson, G. W., Wein, A. J., Raezer, D. M. & Corrier, J. N. (1976) Adrenergic and cholinergic stimulation and blockade of the human bladder base. *Journal of Urology*, **116**, 174.

Blundell & Smith (1968) Faradic stimulation for incontinence. *British Medical Journal*, 431.

Bradley, W. E., Rockswold, G. L., Timm, G. W. & Scott, F. B. (1976) Neurology of micturition, *Journal of Urology*, **115**, 481.

Bradley, W. E., Timm, G. W. & Scott, F. B. (1975) Cystometry, III. Cystometers. *Urology*, **5**, 843.

Brent, L. & Stephens, F. D. (1975) The response of smooth muscle cells in rabbit urinary bladder to outflow obstruction. *Investigative Urology*, **12**, 498.

Brocklehurst, J. C., Armitage, P. & Jouhar, A. J. (1972) Emepronium bromide in urinary incontinence. *Age and Ageing*, **1**, 152.

Brocklehurst, J. C. & Brocklehurst, S. (1977) A study of indwelling catheters in the aged (in press).

Brocklehurst, J. C. (1951) *Incontinence in Old People*. Edinburgh: Livingstone.

Brocklehurst, J. C. (1977) Retention of urine in aged women (in press).

Brocklehurst, J. C., Bee, P., Jones, D. & Palmer, M. (1977) Urinary infection in long-stay geriatric patients *Age and Ageing*.

Brocklehurst, J. C. & Dillane, J. B. (1966a) Studies of the female bladder in old age. 1. Cystometrograms in non-incontinent women. *Gerontologia Clinica*, **8**, 285.

Brocklehurst, J. C. & Dillane, J. B. (1966b) Studies of the female bladder in old age. 2. Cystometrograms in 100 incontinent women. *Gerontologia clinica*, **8**, 306.

Brocklehurst, J. C. & Dillane, J. B. (1967) Studies of the female bladder in old age. 3. Micturating cystograms in incontinent women. *Gerontologia clinica*, **9**, 47.

Brocklehurst, J. C., Dillane, J. B., Griffiths, L. & Fry, J. (1968) The prevalence and symptomatology of urinary infection in an aged population. *Gerontologia clinica*, **10**, 242.

Brocklehurst, J. C., Dillane, J. B., Fry, J. & Armitage, P. (1969) Clinical trial of emepronium bromide in nocturnal frequency of old age. *British Medical Journal*, **ii**, 216.

Brocklehurst, J. C., Fry, J., Griffiths, L. L. & Kalton, G. (1972) Urinary infection and symptoms of dysuria in women age 45–64 years: their relevance to similar findings in the elderly. *Age and Ageing*, **1**, 41.

Brown, A. D. G., Arnold, E. P. & Worth, P. J. L. (1974) The unstable bladder—a study of drug treatment in women (unpublished).

Bruce, A. W., Sira, S. S., Clark, A. F. & Awad, S. A. (1974) The problem of catheter encrustation. *Canadian Medical Association Journal*, **3**, 238.

Buck, A. C., McRae, C. U., Reed, P. I. & Chisholm, G. D. (1974) The diabetic bladder. *Proceedings of the Royal Society of Medicine*, **67**, 81.

Bulmer, D. (1959) The epithelium of the urogenital sinus in female human foetuses. *Journal of Anatomy, (London)*, **93**, 491.

Caldwell, K. P. S. (1967) The treatment of incontinence by electronic implants. *Annals of the Royal College of Surgeons of England*, **41**, 447.

Chiba, R., Imabayashi, K., Igarashi, M., Saside, S., Matsumara, S. & Satake, J. (1967) Experimental studies on the use of ubretid in the field of urology, especially in the neurogenic bladder. *New Remedies and Clinics (Japan)*, **16**, 1368.

Condo, J. (1968) Clinical evaluation of the effects of ubretid on neurogenic bladder dysfunction and high serum–β-glucuronidase activity. *Acta Urology Japon*. **14**, 158.

Cooper, H. H. (1972) *Annals of the Royal College of Surgeons of England*, **51**, 1.

Crisp, J. C., Green, N. A. & Ashken, M. H. (1976) Uro-dynamic studies in the district general hospital. *British Journal of Urology*, **48**, 383.

Diokno, A. C., Coff, S. A. & Bender, L. F. (1974) Peri-urethral striated muscle activity in neurogenic bladder dysfunction. *Journal of Urology*, **112**, 743.

Diokno, A. C., Davis, R. & Lapides, J. (1973) The effect of pelvic nerve stimulation on detrusor contraction. *Investigative Urology*, **11**, 178.

Diokno, A. C., Koss, S. A. & Anderson, W. (1976) Combined cystometry and perineal electromyography in the diagnosis and treatment of neurogenic urinary incontinence. *Journal of Urology*, **115**, 161.

Dobson, P. (1974) *The Management of Incontinence in the Home*. London: Disabled Living Foundation.

Downey, J. W. & Awad, S. A. (1976) The role of neurogenic factors on canine urethral wall tension and urinary continence. *Investigative Urology*, **14**, 143.

Doyle, P. I. & Biscow, C. E. (1976) The effects of drugs and anaesthetic agents on the urinary bladder and sphincter. *British Journal of Urology*, **48**, 329.

Dunn, N., Smith, J. C. & Ardran, G. M. (1974) Prolonged bladder distension as a treatment of urgency and urge incontinence of urine. *British Journal of Urology*, **40**, 645.

Edwards, L. (1976) Electronic Control. In *Incontinence in the Elderly*, ed. Willington, F. L., p. 162. London: Academic Press.

Edwards, L. & Malvern, J. (1974) The urethral pressure profile—theoretical considerations and clinical application. *British Journal of Urology*, **46**, 325.

Edwards, L. & Trott, P. A. (1973) Catheter-induced urethral inflammation. *Journal of Urology*, **110**, 678.

Emmett, J. L., Daut, R. V. & Dunn, J. H. (1948) Role of the external urethral sphincter in the normal bladder and cord bladder. *Journal of Urology*, **59**, 439.

Essenhigh, D. M., Ardran, G. M. & Cope, V. (1968) A study of the bladder outlet in lower urinary tract infections in women. *British Journal of Urology*, **40**, 268.

Farrar, D. J. & Osborne, J. L. (1976) The use of bromocriptine in the treatment of the unstable bladder. *British Journal of Urology*, **48**, 235.

Fox, M., Jarvis, G. L. & Henry, L. (1976) Idiopathic chronic urinary retention in the female. *British Journal of Urology*, **47**, 797.

Geist, S. H. & Salmon, U. J. (1943) The relationship of estrogens to dysuria and incontinence in post-menopausal women. *Journal of Mount Sinai Hospital*, **10**, 208.

Glen, H. E. (1975) Control of incontinence by electrical devices. In *Urinary Incontinence*, ed. Caldwell, K. P. S., p. 89. London: Sector Publishing Ltd.

Gleeson, D. M., Bottaccini, M. R., Reilly, R. J. & Burn, J. C. (1973) Urethral compliance and its role in female voiding dysfunctions. *Investigative Urology*, **11**, 83.

Gosling, J. A. & Dixon, J. S. (1975) The structure and innervation of smooth muscle in the wall of the bladder neck and proximal urethra. *British Journal of Urology*, **47**, 549.

Habshaw, T. & Bennett, J. R. (1972) Ulceration of mouth due to emepronium bromide. *Lancet*, **ii**, 1422.

Harper, W. E. S. & Matz, L. R. (1975) The effect of chlorhexidine irrigation of the bladder in the rat. *British Journal of Urology*, **47**, 539.

Harrison, S. M. (1973) Urinary incontinence of non-neurogenic origin. *Physiotherapy*, **59**, 363.

Harrison, N. W. & Constable, A. R. (1970) Urethral pressure measurement—a modified technique. *British Journal of Urology*, **42**, 229.

Henry, L. & Fox, M. (1971) Histological findings in pseudo-membranous trigonitis. *Journal of Clinical Pathology*, **24**, 605.

Hicks, R. M. (1975) *Biological Reviews*, **50,** 215.
Hodkinson, C. P. (1965) Stress urinary incontinence in the female. *Surgery, Gynecology and Obstetrics,* 595.
Hutch, J. A. (1972) *Anatomy and Physiology of the Bladder, Trigone and Urethra.* Butterworths.
Kegel, A. (1948) Progressive resistance exercise in the functional restoration of the perineal muscles. *American Journal of Obstetrics and Gynecology*, **56,** 238.
Kegel, A. J. (1956) Stress incontinence of urine in women—physiological treatment. *Journal of the International College of Surgeons*, **25,** 487.
Kohler, F. P. & Morales, P. A. (1968) Cystometric evaluation of flavoxate-hydrochloride in normal and neurogenic bladders. *Journal of Urology*, **100,** 729.
Langworthy, O. R., Kolb, L. C. & Lewis, L. G. (1940) *Physiology of Micturition.* Baltimore: Williams and Wilkins Co.
Lapides, J., Diokno, A., Goulde, F. R. & Lowe, B. S. (1976) Further observations on self-catheterisation. *Journal of Urology*, **116,** 169.
Lapides, J. (1964) Urecholine regime for rehabilitating the atonic bladder. *Journal of Urology*, **91,** 658.
Lapides, J., Diokno, A. C., Lowe, B. S. & Kalish, M. D. (1974) Follow-up on unsterile intermittent self-catheterisation. *Journal of Urology*, **111,** 184.
Macmillan, S. A. (1972) Bacteriuria of elderly women in hospital—occurrence and drug resistance. *Lancet*, **ii,** 452.
Mandelstan, D. (1976) *Incontinence.* London: Disabled Living Foundation.
Mayo, M. E., Lloyd-Davis, R. W., Shuttleworth, K. E. D. & Tighe, J. R. (1973) The human damaged detrusor-functional and electron-microscopic changes in disease. *British Journal of Urology*, **45,** 116.
McLennan, F. C. (1939) *The Neurogenic Bladder.* Springfield, Illinois: Charles C. Thomas.
Meisels, A. (1966) The menopause—a cytohormonal study. *Acta Cytologica*, **10,** 49.
Milne, J. S., Williamson, J., Maule, M. M. & Wallace, E. T. (1972) Urinary symptoms in older people. *Modern Geriatrics*, **2,** 198.
Montgomery, E. (1974) *Regaining Bladder Control.* Bristol: John Wright.
Moore, T. & Schofield, P. N. (1967) The treatment of stress incontinence by maximal perineal electrical stimulation. *British Medical Journal*, **iii,** 150.
Nergardh, A. (1975) Autonomic receptor functions in the lower urinary tract: a survey of recent experimental results. *Journal of Urology*, **113,** 180.
Niijima, T. & Asano, M. (1967) clinical appraisal of ubretid a new anti-cholinesterase inhibitor, in urology. *Acta Urology Japan*, **13,** 423.
Orikasa, S., Koyanagi, T., Motomura, M., Kudo, T., Togashi, M. & Tsuji, I. (1976) Experience with non-sterile intermittent self-catheterisation. *Journal of Urology*, **115,** 141.
Packham, D. A. (1971) The epithelial lining of the female trigone and urethra. *British Journal of Urology*, **43,** 201.
Parvinen, M., Sourander, L. B. & Vuorinen, P. (1965) Cystographic studies of old women. *Gerontologia clinica*, **7,** 343.
Radej, M., Hitrec, V., Krivec, O., Kovacic, M., Parazajder, J. & Pavletic, M. (1976) Functional and tonometrical investigation of bladder and urethral in patients with stress incontinence. *Journal of Urology*, **115,** 551.
Randall, N. J. (1975) A new uroflow meter for routine clinical use. *Biomedical Engineering*, **10,** 21.
Raz, S. & Smith, R. B. (1976) External sphincter spasticity syndrome in female patients. *Journal of Urology*, **115,** 443.
Roberts, M. & Smith, P. (1968) Non-malignant obstruction of the female urethra. *British Journal of Urology*, **40,** 694.
Rohner, T. J., Raeger, D. M., Wein, A. J. & Schernberg, H. W. (1971) Contractile responses of dog bladder neck. *Journal of Urology*, **105,** 657.
Rutte, B. von & Delnon, I. (1968) Die Urethralzytologie und ihre bedeutung zur Diagnose hormonal bedingter miktionsstorungen. *Praxis*, **16,** 555.
Sadoughi, N., Razvi, N., Ablin, R. J. & Bush, I. M. (1975) The effects of digitalis on the bladder neck in man. *Journal of Urology*, **113,** 178.
Shand, D. G., O'Grady, F., Nimmon, C. C. & Katel, W. R. (1970) Relation between residual urine volume and response to treatment of urinary infection. *Lancet*, **i,** 1305.
Smith, P. (1972) Age changes in the female urethra. *British Journal of Urology*, **42,** 667.
Smith, P. (1971) Incontinence pads containing carboxymethylcellulose. *Practitioner*, **207,** 111.
Smith, P., Roberts, M. & Slade, N. (1970) Urinal symptoms following hysterectomy. *British Journal of Urology*, **42,** 3.
Stanton, S. L. (1973) A comparison of emepronium bromide and flavoxate hydrochloride in the treatment of urinary incontinence. *Journal of Urology*, **110.** 529.

Stanton, S. L. (1972) Urethral incontinence in women. *Proceedings of the Royal Society of Medicine*, **65,** 829.

Stolle, P. Vaginal cytology: Date and volume not available.

Strauss, B. S. & Blaufox, M. D. (1970) Estimation of residual urine and urine flow rates without urethral catheterisation. *Journal of Nuclear Medicine*, **II,** 81.

Streitz, J. M. (1963) Squamous epithelium in the female trigone. *Journal of Urology*, **90,** 62.

Strouthidis, T. M., Mankikar, G. D. & Irvine, R. E. (1972) Ulceration of mouth due to emepronium bromide. *Lancet*.

Sundin, T. & Peterson, I. (1975) Cystometry and simultaneous electromyography from the striated urethral and anal sphincters and from the levator ani. *Investigative Urology*, **13,** 40.

Tanagho, E. A., Smith, D. R. & Meyers, F. J. (1968) The trigone—anatomical and physiological considerations (in relation to the bladder neck). *Journal of Urology*, **100,** 633.

Tanner, E. R. (1969) Pelvic muscle dysfunction in urinary incontinence. *Physiotherapy*, 372.

Thompson, J. (1964) Cystometry in investigation of urinary incontinence. *Current Achievements in Geriatrics*. London: Cassell.

Tscholl, R., Tetamanti, F. & Worsdorfer, O. (1976) The urethral profile recorded by means of CO_2 perfusion at high flow rates. *British Journal of Urology*, **48,** 337.

Tyler, D. E. (1962) Stratified squamous epithelium in vesical trigone and urethral. Findings correlated with the menstrual cycle and age. *American Journal of Anatomy*, **111,** 319.

Tulloch, A. G. S. (1974) The vascular contribution to intra-urethral pressure. *British Journal of Urology*, **46,** 659.

Wastling, G. (1972) A genito-urinary nursing scheme. *Nursing Times*, **69,** 1128.

Wastling, G. (1974) Long-term catheterisation. *Nursing Times*, **71,** 17.

Welsh Hospital Board, Supplies Division (1972) *A Report on the Study and Evaluative Trial of an Incontinence Garment*.

Wessen, M. B. (1920) Studies of the trigone. *Journal of Urology*, **4,** 279.

Whiteside, C. G. & Arnold, E. P. (1975) Persistent primary enuresis. *British Medical Journal*, **i,** 364.

Whitfield, H. M., Doyle, P. T., Mayle, M. E. & Poopalsingham, N. (1976) The effect of adrenergic blocking drugs on outflow resistance. *British Journal of Urology*, **47,** 823.

Whitfield, H. M. & Mayo, M. E. (1975) Prolonged bladder distension in the treatment of the unstable bladder. *British Journal of Urology*, **47,** 635.

Willington, F. L. (1975) Management of urinary incontinence. In *Urinary Incontinence*, ed. Caldwell, p. 129. London: Sector Publishing Ltd.

Willington, F. L. (1976) Hygienic methods of management of incontinence. In *Incontinence in the Elderly*, ed. Willington, F. L., p. 227. London: Academic Press.

Wilson, T. S. (1948) Incontinence of urine in the aged. *Lancet*, **ii,** 374.

Woodburne, R. T. (1968) Anatomy of the bladder—bladder outlet. *Journal of Urology*, **100,** 474.

Youngblood, V. H., Tomlin, E. M., Williams, J. O. & Kimilstein, P. (1958) Exfoliative cytology of the senile female urethra. *Journal of Urology*, **79,** 110.

Zuckerman, S. (1940) The histogenesis of tissues sensitive to oestrogens. *Biological Reviews*. **15,** 231.

3. Biochemical changes in the normal ageing brain and in dementia

David M. Bowen   Alan N. Davison

Senile dementia can be regarded as a 'major killer' (Katzman, 1976). It is unclear whether this disorder is a distinct disease entity or whether it represents an exacerbation of normal ageing. We therefore devote this section to a review of neural systems that are vulnerable in normal ageing. The biochemical findings emphasised are those that give information about quantitative changes in neural cell number, subcellular structure and defects in synaptic transmission.

The following abbreviations will be used:

NFD—neurofibrillary degeneration
GAD—glutamate decarboxylase
CAT—choline acetyl transferase
AChE—acetylcholinesterase
TH—tyrosine hydroxylase
AAD—aromatic amino acid decarboxylase
MAO—monoamine oxidase
CNP—adenosine-2′3′-cyclic nucleotide-3′-phosphohydrolase
5HT—serotonin
ACh—acetylcholine
AII—angiotensin II
S100, 14.3.2 and NS6 are soluble acidic proteins enriched in brain.

VULNERABLE SYSTEMS IN THE NORMAL BRAIN

Atrophy of the brain, enlarged ventricles and thickening of the leptomeninges are common findings in aged humans. In animals there appears to be a decrease in the extracellular space (Bondareff, 1976) and a general correlation between decreasing numbers of cells in the brain and increasing age.

Atrophy of the brain

The mean weight of the male brain drops from 1400 g at age 30 by approximately 5 per cent at the age of 70, by 10 per cent at age 80 and by 20 per cent by 90 years. There is histological evidence of some loss of neurones, for example, Purkinje cells from the cerebellar cortex and probably also cortical neurones; but in general this loss is minor and in other areas of the brain fall-out of nerve cells has not been unequivocally observed.

Psychomotor function

Deterioration in psychomotor function with advancing age may be a function of the quality of neuropil (Scheibel and Scheibel, 1975). Changes in evoked potential of senescent individuals correlate with shrinkage of the brain stem and of the ventricular core. Gradual decline in homoeostatic stability during ageing is associated more directly with structural and functional changes in the brain and neuroendocrines, e.g. salt and water balance and the regulation of cerebral blood pressure under central control of angiotensin II (Barker, 1976).

Neuronal changes

In the elderly human brain some morphological changes are seen in neurones, particularly in the neocortex and hippocampus. These include neurofibrillary degeneration (NFD), granulovacuolar degeneration and the accumulation of insoluble lipofuscin granules (Tomlinson and Henderson, 1976). Apart from the deposition of lipofuscin these changes are not generally apparent in animals.

Blood flow and energy metabolism

In ageing healthy human subjects, slow decline in cognitive ability is accompanied by small changes in blood flow. Between the ages of 30 and 90 there is little reduction in metabolic rate. There is no apparent difference in cerebral oxygen consumption between normal young people and non-arteriosclerotic elderly subjects. In older subjects cerebral glucose consumption may be reduced to about 80 per cent of that found in younger people. Glucose is the sole substrate for the normal young adult brain but in the elderly there is increased utilisation of ketone bodies (Sokoloff, 1976), accounting for the difference in oxygen consumption. There is abundant evidence that in non-anoxic brain tissue the blood flow is controlled mainly by the functional activity of the neurone (Ingvar, 1976). Using radioactive xenon clearance it has been demonstrated that, in the resting state, cerebral blood flow is highest in the premotor and frontal regions and lowest in the temporal and occipital areas. Significant changes in blood flow to the dominant hemisphere occur in response to functional demand. For example, problem solving increases the blood supply to the premotor and frontal regions.

NEUROCHEMICAL STUDIES IN ANIMALS

Animals as a model of the human brain

A myriad of developmental and ageing studies have utilised brain from small laboratory animals. These, arguably, do little to advance our knowledge of certain aspects of the human ageing brain, for there is a great increase in neocortical development in man and apes as compared to experimental animals. This evolutionary development led Broca to call the cerebral mantle 'la partie intelligente'. There is, however, a degree of evolutionary stability in the limbic system, striatum and hypothalamic-pituitary-adrenal axis. Therefore biochemical data obtained using these regions from lower animals are thought to be relevant to the mechanisms of the human brain which control human behaviour, emotion, movement and homoeostasis during ageing. For example, in senescent mice the metabolic turnover of catecholamine neurotransmitters is reduced in the hypothalamus and striatum (Finch, 1976).

Another problem encountered when using animals as a model of man's brain is their greatly differing life-spans. In mice the brain weight is maximal at about 90 days, but the mouse continues to grow slowly throughout life. Moreover, the life-span varies from strain to strain. The brain weight of man and of rhesus monkey reach their maximum at about

12.5 and 4 years respectively (Himwich, 1973). Since the recorded maximum longevity of *Macaco mulatta* is 31 years (Ordy, Kaach and Brizzee, 1975) it appears that the brains of man and monkey reach maturity at approximately the same relative age in development. There are, however, no neurochemical data for monkeys over the age of 16 years.

BIOCHEMICAL INDICES OF BRAIN STRUCTURE IN HUMANS

The few original papers dealing with the ageing human brain have been repeatedly reviewed (e.g. Perez and Moore, 1970; Ordy et al, 1975; Davis and Himwich, 1975). One serious inadequacy of almost all previous studies of the biochemistry of 'normal' human brain is that the specimens which were analysed were not assessed for possible histological abnormality.

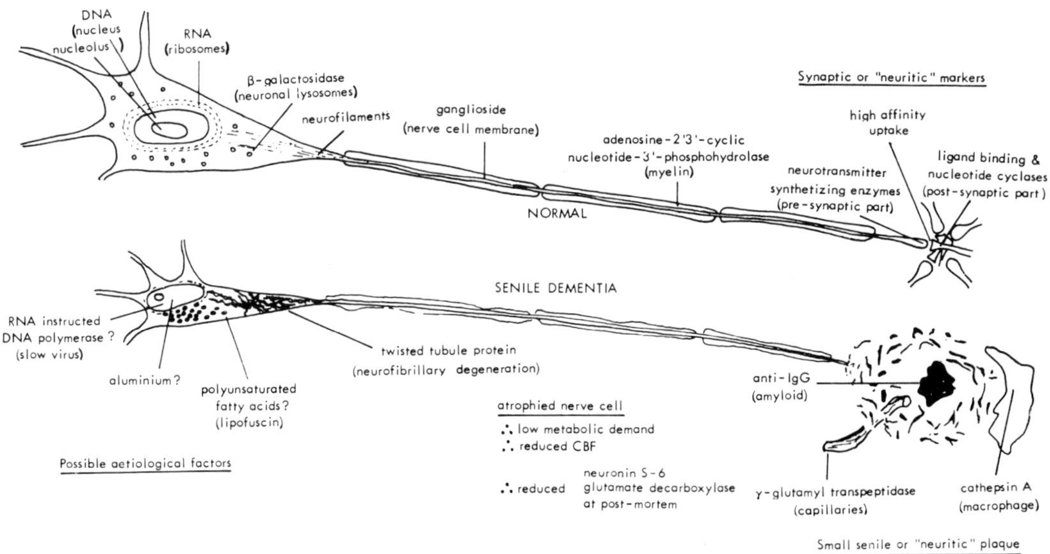

Fig. 3.1 Biochemical indices of senile brain degeneration

Does neuronal loss occur in normal ageing?

The interpretation of biochemical changes detected in brain postmortem requires morphological examination of all brain regions, details of clinical history and the autopsy findings in other organs (Bowen et al, 1976a). An example of the difficulty is that a study of whole brain showed a 25 per cent loss of total lipid and a 28 per cent loss of protein by 90 years of age (Ordy et al, 1975). One might conclude that neural cells were lost at a mean rate of approximately 0.3 per cent/year. However, total ganglioside NANA content per wet weight of frontal cortex measured as a tentative index of nerve cell membranes (Fig. 3.1) remains constant throughout life (for reference see Bowen, Smith and Davison, 1973). This finding suggests that the relative proportion of neurones to glia remains essentially unaltered throughout life.

There is evidence that intracellular autophagocytic vacuoles (lysosomes) are converted to lipofuscin (Bowen, Davison and Ramsey, 1974). Polyunsaturated fatty acids are particularly susceptible to auto-oxidation which might be responsible for increased deposition of the ageing pigment. This could be relevant because polyunsaturated fatty acid content seems to be increased in atrophic brain. However, whether or not these changes are related to neuronal loss is not clear; for although increasing amounts of lipofuscin are found in the neurones of the inferior olive from birth, there is no age-related loss of neurones from this region (Brody, 1976).

Glial change

Microscopic studies by Cragg and others on human and animal brain show no changes with ageing in the ratio of synapses to neuronal perikarya, or of astrocytes to oligodendrocytes (Bowen and Davison, 1976). This conclusion is not at variance with the findings that there is an apparent increase with advancing years in the glial cell population of the brain

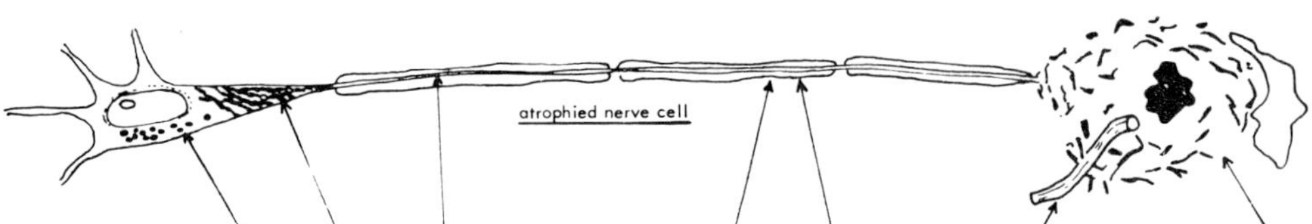

Diagnostic group	neuronal loss (mean score)	β-galactosidase (% reduction)	NFD (mean score)	ganglioside (% reduction)	glutamate decarboxylase (% reduction)	nucleotide phosphohydrolase (% reduction)	myelin loss (mean score)	γ-glutamyl transpeptidase (% reduction)	choline esterase (% reduction)	senile plaques (mean score)
Control	0.2	0	0	0	0	0	nd	0	0	0.2
Senile dementia	1.7	48[b]	0.7	34[b]	74[d]	37[c]	1.0	0	52[a]	2.0
"Vascular dementia"	1.8	33	1.3	46[c]	60	32[a]	1.8	0	nd	2.3

[a,b,c] P at least < 0.05, 0.02, 0.01, respectively; [d] significantly different from both other groups (P at least < 0.025).

Results, except for GTP and GAD activities in frontal cortex, are for temporal lobe.

Fig. 3.2 Biochemical and morphological changes in temporal lobe from cases of organic 'senile-type' dementia (Bowen et al, 1977a). The morphological changes were assessed using a scale: 0, 1, 2 and 3—zero, slight, moderate, severe. The biochemical changes are calculated from data expressed per temporal lobe. 'Vascular dementia' is mixed senile and vascular dementias

i.e. increased density of the glial cells can be caused by shrinkage of the neuronal perikarya (Lange et al, 1976) or by a decrease in cortical dendritic density, both of which occur in the ageing brain. There is evidence that the microglia double in number in old age, even though they are a very minor component of normal brain.

NEUROCHEMICAL STUDIES

In an attempt to establish which neural elements are most affected by ageing we measured the activity of seven enzymes and the concentration of various substances in human brain. Analyses were made on the entire temporal lobe in order to reduce errors due to uneven sampling, oedema, or water loss. The results on homogenic samples were expressed per lobe and were corrected for lobe weight differences between the sexes, so that estimates could be made of cellular change.

Linear regression analysis of the data for lobes from control cases (Fig. 3.2) aged 50 to 100 years, showed that with the exception of the RNA/DNA ratio (see page 54) the potential indices of total nerve and glial cell number did not change with increasing age. However, the concentration of substances which were thought to be 'markers' of the synapse and axons, i.e. glutamate decarboxylase (GAD), acetylcholinesterase (AChE), and adenosine-2′3′-cyclic nucleotide-3′-phosphohydrolase (CNP) tended to decrease with advancing age (Fig. 3.3).

NEUROTRANSMITTERS

Acetylcholine (ACh), γ-aminobutyric acid (GABA), noradrenaline (NA) and possibly serotonin (5HT) are important transmitters in the cortex.

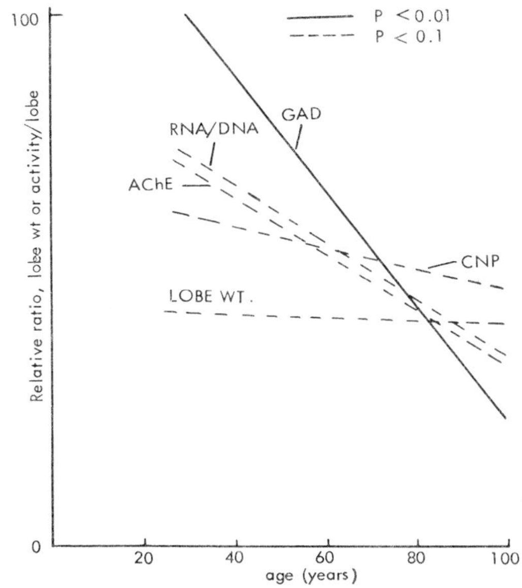

Fig. 3.3 Unit changes in biochemical constituents (vertical axis) as a function of age at death in temporal lobes from control cases (Bowen et al, 1977b). The best straight line from the data is shown. The solid line has a correlation of $P < 0.01$

Acetylcholine

The synthesis of ACh is catalysed by choline acetyltransferase (CAT) which is concentrated in the striatum (Table 3.1). CAT activity in the brain may decline with increasing age particularly during the first five decades of life (Fig. 3.4) although it is not known if there is any change in the ACh content of the brain. From studies in the mouse it appears that the rate of transport of CAT from the site of enzyme synthesis in the neuronal perikarya to the nerve endings, declines by the time the brain weight has matured (Fig. 3.4). The density of muscarinic cholinergic receptor binding sites decreases with increasing age (James and Kanungo, 1976) as judged by the binding of atropine to synaptosomal fractions prepared from cerebral cortices of rats.

In human cortex there are indications that, at the age of 60 to 70 years, receptor binding also declines (White et al, 1977) as measured by a similar technique. When ACh receptors in healthy young human subjects were blocked with scopolamine, the functional deficits mimicked those seen in old age (Fig. 3.5). This suggests that the decreased ability of old people to remember recent events is related to a deficit in the cholinergic system.

Table 3.1 Regional distribution of indices of centrally acting peptides and specific types of neurones

	Peptide markers		
Brain region	Angiotensin converting activity[a] (human)	Enkephalin[b] (rabbit)	Opiate receptors[c] (human)
Neocortex			
Frontal	25	5	48
Occipital	10		10
Cerebellum	6	0	<6
Hippocampus	12	8	39
Amygdala	16	—	148
Hypothalamus	20	30	77
Caudate nucleus	100	100	100

	Markers of cholinergic neurones				
			Choline acetyltransferase		
Brain region	Receptor binding[d] (QNB) (monkey)	Choline uptake[d] (monkey)	(human)[e]	(monkey)[d]	AChE[e] (human)
Neocortex					
Frontal	44	4	5	6	10
Occipital	58	3	4	4	10
Cerebellum	13	4	4	1	25
Hippocampus	50	15	8	17	14
Amygdala	50	—	20	33	25
Hypothalamus	24	23	7	18	23
Caudate nucleus	100	100	100	100	100

	Markers of other neurones		
Brain region	Tyrosine hydroxylase (TH)[e] (human)	Aromatic acid decarboxylase (AAD)[e] (human)	Glutamate decarboxylase (GAD)[e] (human)
Neocortex			
Frontal	tr.	tr.	165
Occipital	tr.	tr.	128
Cerebellum	tr.	tr.	99
Hippocampus	23	tr.	66
Amygdala	11	70	59
Hypothalamus	59	82	141
Caudate nucleus	100	100	100

Activity or concentration as percentage of that in caudate; tr., trace
References: [a]Poth et al, 1975; [b]Hughes, 1975; [c]Kuhar et al, 1973; [d]Yamamura et al, 1974; [e]McGeer and McGeer, 1976b

Aromatic biogenic amines

The rate-controlling enzymes for NA and 5HT synthesis are respectively tyrosine (TH) and tryptophan hydroxylases. The precursor amino acids are derived from the blood. The concentration of NA and the activity of two of the NA synthesising enzymes (TH and aromatic amino acid decarboxylase (AAD)), decrease with advancing age. According to most studies, the activity of the catabolic enzyme monoamine oxidase (MAO) increases with increasing age (Fig. 3.6).

γ-Aminobutyric acid

GABA synthesis is catalysed by the pyridoxal phosphate-requiring enzyme GAD. The apoenzyme has been highly purified, allowing electron microscopic immunolocalisation studies to be carried out. These show that, like CAT, the enzyme is located in nerve endings. The GABA content and the GAD activity are more evenly distributed through

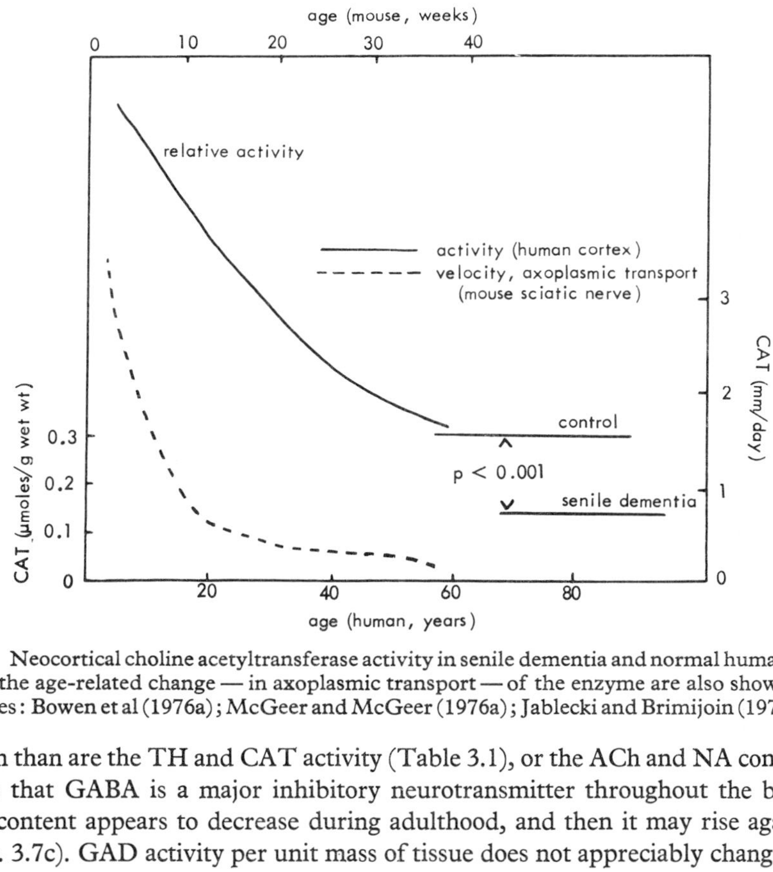

Fig. 3.4 Neocortical choline acetyltransferase activity in senile dementia and normal human brain. Data for the age-related change — in axoplasmic transport — of the enzyme are also shown. References: Bowen et al (1976a); McGeer and McGeer (1976a); Jablecki and Brimijoin (1975)

the brain than are the TH and CAT activity (Table 3.1), or the ACh and NA content. This suggests that GABA is a major inhibitory neurotransmitter throughout the brain. The GABA content appears to decrease during adulthood, and then it may rise again in late life (Fig. 3.7c). GAD activity per unit mass of tissue does not appreciably change after the age of about 50 years (Fig. 3.7a). However, activity decreases during the first five decades, particularly in the thalamus (McGeer and McGeer, 1976a).

Centrally acting peptides

The central neurophysiological action of some peptides has been reviewed by Barker (1976). The vasodilator substance-P (Fig. 3.8) is one such peptide. This compound may be important in Parkinson's disease, for it is differentially distributed in the spinal cord (Cuello, Polak and Pearse, 1976) and in the regions of the substantia nigra, the reticular part containing almost 100 times more than the cortex (Brownstein et al, 1976). Vasopressin, another neuroactive peptide (Fig. 3.8) with vasodilator activity, is synthesised in the perikarya of nerve cells in the anterior hypothalamus. The precursor of another active peptide, angiotensin II (Fig. 3.8), which has vasoconstrictor activity, occurs in the blood. Human brain contains the enzymes necessary for synthesising angiotensin from the precursor (Poth, Heath and Ward, 1975). Cathepsin A (an exopeptide acting at acid pH values) inactivates angiotensin and may also actively destroy leu-enkephalin as judged by

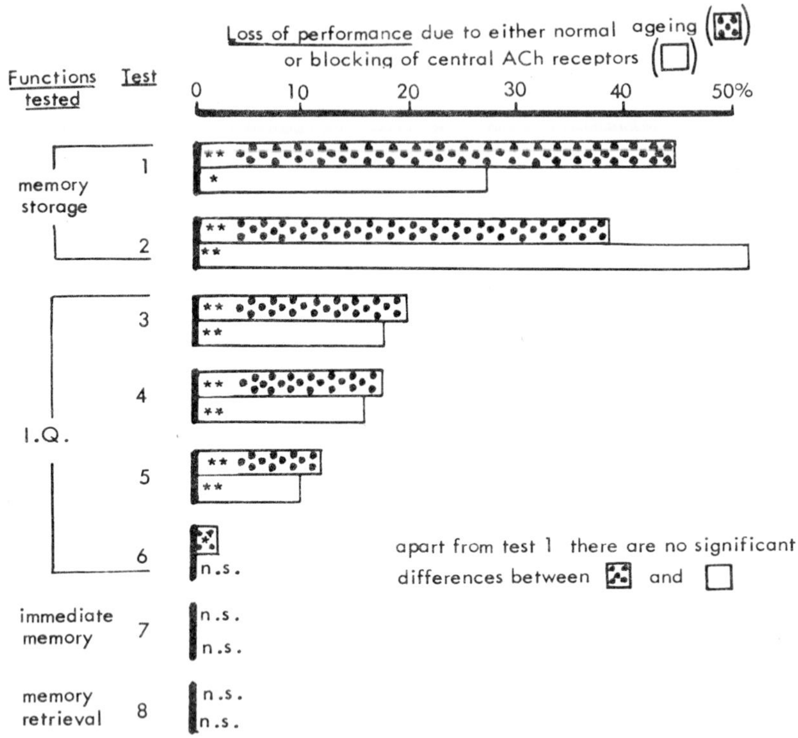

Fig. 3.5 Pharmacological evidence that the cholinergic system is involved in human age-related memory loss. Modified from Drachman and Leavitt (1974). Loss due to *normal ageing* is the performance of subjects with a mean age of 22 (normal controls) compared with the performance of subjects of mean age 67 years. Loss due to *blocking of ACh receptors* is the performance of normal controls before and after the administration of scopolamine (selective blocking of peripheral receptors had no effect on performance). Asterisks inside bars identify the level of significance of the loss of performance: $*P = 0.05$ or $**P = 0.01$ and n.s. is non-significant. Apart from test 1 there are no significant differences between aged and scopolamine treated subjects

the rapid rate at which the enzyme acts on a synthetic substrate (Grynbaum and Marks, 1976). In normal human brain cathepsin A, like other acid hydrolases, is enriched in neuronal lysosomes (Bowen et al, 1973, 1977a). The proportion of non-lysosomal bound activity may increase with advancing years (Bowen and Radin, 1969). In view of the probable association in diseased brain of cathepsin A activity, macrophages (Fig. 3.1, Bowen and Davison, 1974) and 'senile' morphological changes (Bowen et al, 1977a) it is of interest that microgliomatosis can present with organic dementia and hypopituitarism (Fig. 3.9).

Interaction of the cholinergic system

Neurophysiological data, obtained using the subfornical organ (part of the hypothalamus), and recent neurochemical results suggest that angiotensin may act as a neurotransmitter (or modulator) both in specific *octapeptidergic* and in cholinergic central neurones (Phillips and Felix, 1976; Bennett, Arregui and Snyder, 1976). In contrast to the action of angiotensin, morphine-like drugs are often anticholinergic. There is a combination of anticholinergic and narcotic-analgesic factors in sleep (Byck, 1976). In human cortex there is some correspondence between the regional distribution of putative binding sites (opiate receptors) for enkephalin (Hughes, 1975) and the C-fragment of β-lipotropin (Bradbury, Smyth and Snell, 1976) (Fig. 3.8) and angiotensin-converting enzyme activity (Table 3.1).

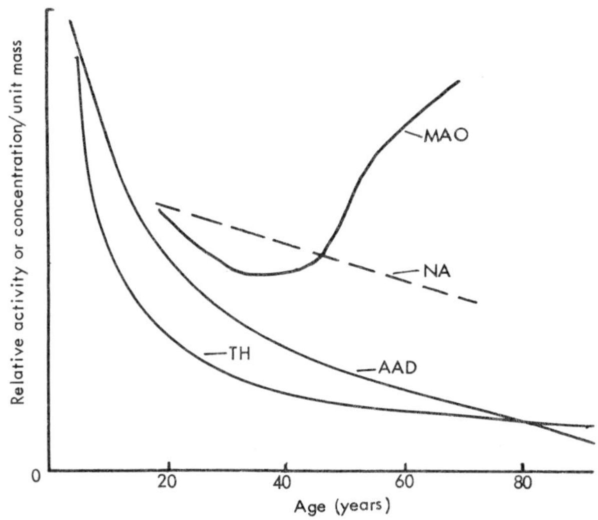

Fig. 3.6 Age-related cnanges in the metabolism of noradrenaline (NA) in human brain. McGeer and McGeer (1975); Bowen et al (1976a); Robinson et al (1972). Brain regions: putamen for tyrosine hydroxylase (TH), caudate nucleus for aromatic amino acid decarboxylase (AAD) and hindbrain for monoamine oxidases (MAO)

Limbic system and memory

Opiate receptor-binding sites may be concentrated in the limbic system (Kuhar, Pert and Snyder, 1973). Vasopressin acts in the mid-brain limbic system, including the hippocampus, facilitating the consolidation of memory and the development of resistance to narcotic analgesics (Wimersma-Greidanus and Wied, 1977). Autophagocytic vacuole-like granulovacuolar degeneration in the hippocampus (Bowen et al, 1974) occurs characteristically in senile dementia. Although Broca implied that the limbic system had functions other than those related to smell, it has only recently been appreciated that the temporal components of the limbic system are important in memory (Corsellis, 1976), where memory mechanisms are localised by other parts of the brain (for discussion see Bowen and Davison, 1976).

BIOCHEMICAL CHANGES IN DEMENTIA

In this section three types of dementia are discussed. 'Vascular dementia', the Diagnostic Division 0:1 of Corsellis (1962), is characterised by the presence of severe focal atheroma

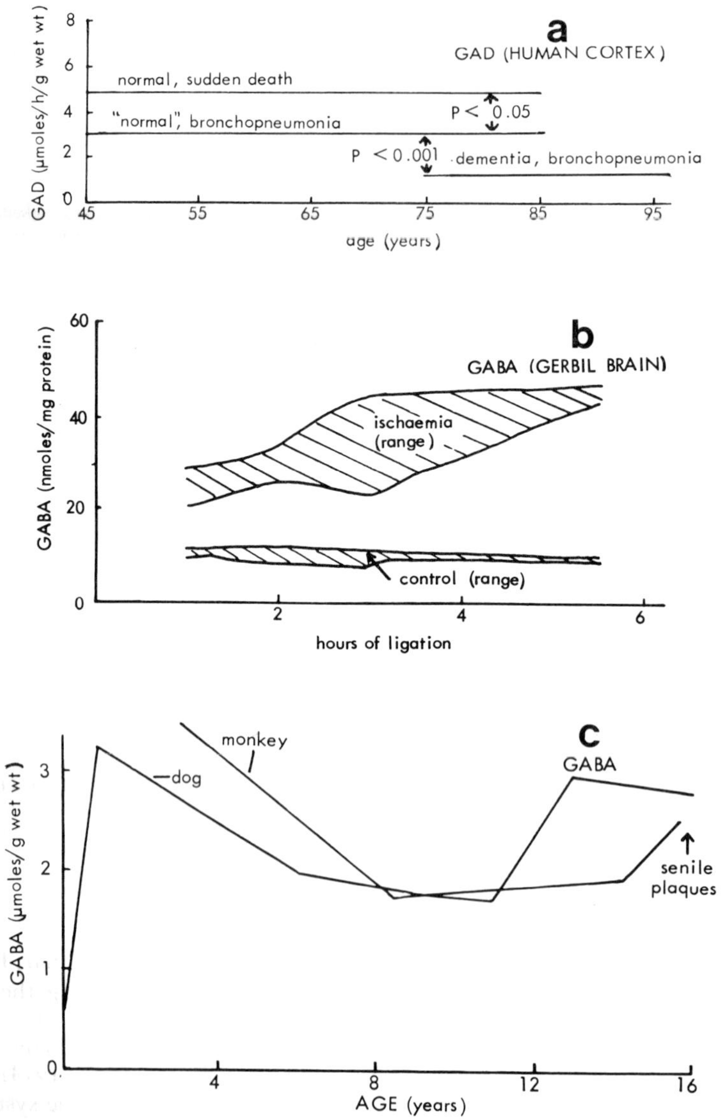

Fig. 3.7 Metabolism of γ-aminobutyric acid (GABA) in normal ageing, senile dementia and ischaemia. References: (a) Bowen et al (1976a); (b) Lust et al (1975); (c) tissue content of GABA for animal species in which senile plaques are present (Davis and Himwich, 1975)

and arteriosclerosis. In other brains there are concomitant diffuse changes of the senile type (atrophy, senile plaques and NFD) with dementia. Patients with this brain pathology are described as having mixed senile and vascular dementia (or Diagnostic Division 0:3; Corsellis, 1962). The senile form of degeneration may also occur in the absence of significant

Asp-Arg-Val-Tyr-Ile -His-Pro-Phe

angiotensin

Arg-Pro-Lys-Pro-Gln-Gln-Phe-Phe-Gly-Leu-Met (NH_2)

substance-P

Cys-Tyr-Phe-Gln-Asn-Cys-Pro-Arg-Gly (NH_2)

vasopressin

Tyr-Gly-Gly-Phe-Met (or Leu)

enkephalin

Tyr-Gly-Gly-Phe-Met-(21 residues)-His-Lys-Lys-Gly-Gln

C-fragment of β-lipotropin

Fig. 3.8 Structure of some centrally acting peptides

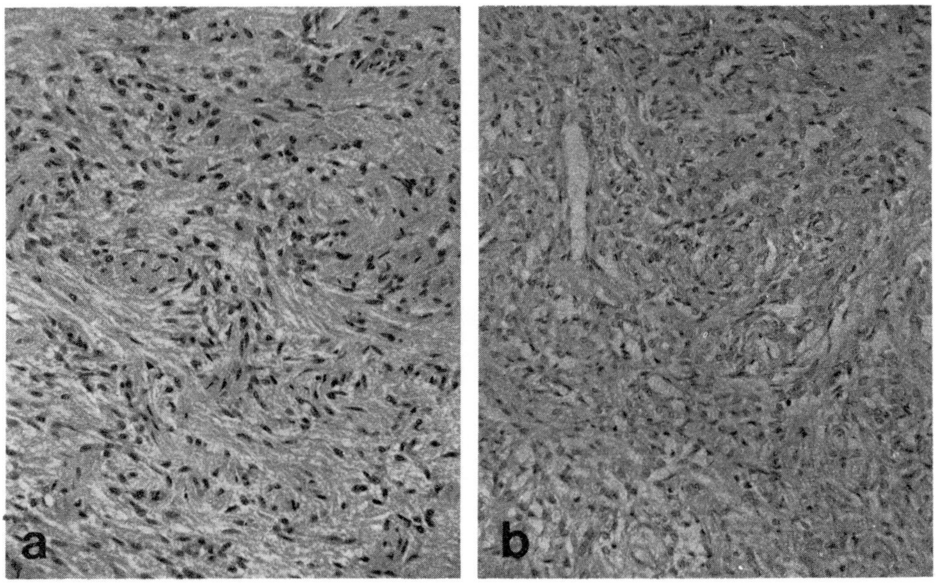

Fig. 3.9 Neurohypophysis of a normal subject (a) compared with that of the demented case (b). Note the densely cellular appearance of (b) which is due to loss of hypothalamoneuropophyseal nerve fibres. Photographs were kindly donated by Professor Duchen and Dr Treip. They are taken from Duchen and Treip (1969)

small vessel disease. In patients over the age of 70 years this condition is known as senile dementia (Diagnostic Division 0:2; Corsellis, 1962). Patients with either senile dementia or mixed senile and vascular dementia are referred to as cases of organic 'senile-type' dementia.

Evolution of 'vascular dementia'

The arteries of the brain respond to a persistent rise in luminal blood pressure by hypertrophy of the muscular medial coat with elongation of the arteries to produce a 'spiralling' effect. This increases with advancing age in arteries, arterioles, capillaries and venules throughout the whole thickness of the cerebral cortex and the white matter (Fang, 1976). The artery becomes separated from the tissue by a fluid-filled channel, and this results in a loss of sensitivity of the artery to changes in oxygen. An inappropriate metabolism of at least one centrally acting peptide, angiotensin II, might contribute to this process by promoting idiopathic hypertension (Barker, 1976). In some subjects this physiological process is masked by focal atheroma and arteriosclerosis. When these changes are severe in elderly people, dementia may occur.

Cerebral blood flow in dementia

In patients described as having 'chronic brain syndrome and psychosis' the early studies of Kety demonstrated significant reduction in cerebral oxygen and glucose consumption (Sokoloff, 1975). Measurement of cerebral blood flow by the intracarotid radioactive xenon technique (Hachinski et al, 1974) showed significant loss of the fast-clearing tissues (largely grey matter), in multi-infarct (i.e. patients that presumably correspond to those in Diagnostic Division 0:1 and 0:3) and Alzheimer's dementias. However, the weighted mean blood flow of 49 ml/100 g/min in the Alzheimer group was not significantly different from the normal figure of 56, but in multi-infarct dementia a highly significant difference in blood flow of 36 ml/100 g/min was seen. This reduction is probably due to the presence of an appreciable proportion of infarcted tissue since the mean flow rate is calculated from the proportion of fast- and slow-clearing tissues and their respective flow rates. In later stages of senile dementia there is a substantial reduction in cerebral flow changes (Ingvar and Gustafson, 1970), presumably related to brain atrophy.

Changes in blood flow on challenge

There is evidence (Ingvar, Risberg and Schwartz Martin, 1975) of subnormal function of the association cortex in Alzheimer's disease and low pressure hydrocephalus. The blood flow to the grey matter was significantly reduced, especially in the occipital-parieto-temporal regions. The augmentation of flow in demented patients in the association areas during attempted activation by reading and psychological tests was less than normal; and in some cases the blood flow was diminished. Such alterations in blood flow are related to the vasodilation induced by carbon dioxide, which is released by the increased metabolic activity of the neurones (Siesjö, 1977). Impaired ability to learn a complex task and defective short-term memory were observed under hypoxic conditions when the alveolar $P\text{O}_2$ was reduced to 55 to 60 mmHg. These defects were exaggerated by hypocapnia and were improved when CO_2 was administered.

Effect of 'hypoxia' on transmitters

Experimental ischaemia. After ligation of the carotid artery in the Mongolian gerbil the GABA content increased in the damaged hemisphere (Fig. 3.7b). Bowen et al (1976b) showed that energy-dependent GABA uptake into synaptosomes and GAD activity were particularly affected. Choline uptake (Goodhardt et al, 1976) and CAT activity (Bowen and Davison, 1976) were relatively less affected. The concentration of neuronin S6 (NS6), a soluble acidic protein that is enriched in brain, was also decreased in ischaemia. The amounts of soluble S100 and the brain specific proteins 14.3.2 were not affected.

In senile dementia. The NS6 content and the GAD activity but not the CAT activity were reduced in specimens of cortex from 'normal' patients who died of bronchopneumonia (Fig. 3.7a). The reduction was even greater in cases of senile dementia. These findings were consistent with the view that cerebral blood flow is reduced, at least terminally in senile dementia.

Cerebral lysosomes are thought to be relatively resistant to 'lysis' during ischaemia (Clendenon et al, 1971). Thus, terminal phenomena may not explain the marked increase in the proportion of AII inactivating enzyme (cathepsin A) and β-galactosidase activity in the cytoplasm or cytosol of homogenates of the brains of patients dying with senile dementia (Bowen, Smith and Davison, 1973).

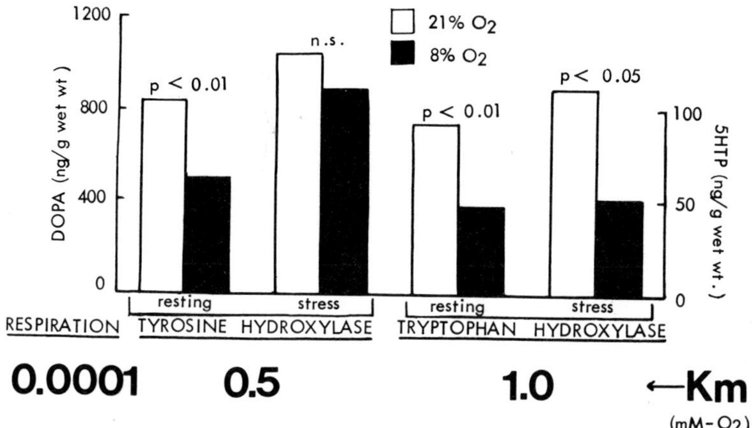

Fig. 3.10 Some environmental factors affecting the synthesis of aromatic biogenic amines in a noradrenaline dominated brain region. Rats were pretreated with an inhibitor of aromatic amino acid decarboxylase and then were placed in chambers of appropriate oxygen content for 45 min (resting). Some of the animals received electrical foot shocks during the 45 min period (stress). References: Brown, Snider and Carlsson (1974); Bachelard (1976)

Low oxygen tension

The aromatic biogenic amine hydroxylation reactions, catalysed by TH and tryptophan hydroxylase, utilise molecular oxygen. As judged by the Km values (Fig. 3.10) these enzymes show a far lower affinity for oxygen than do the enzymes associated with brain respiration. Consequently, a lowering of oxygen tension is more likely to affect the synthesis of NA, dopamine and 5HT than of ATP. Thus, in resting animals, hypoxia retards the formation of DOPA and 5-hydroxytryptophan (5HTP, Fig. 3.10) while in normoxic animals, stress, which presumably causes increased neuronal activity, stimulates the synthesis of both compounds. However, when animals are stressed and made hypoxic only, 5HTP synthesis is depressed. This demonstrates that the activation of catecholamine systems by stress renders them resistant to hypoxia. This adaptive mechanism may be nullified or modified in old age, with the result that vulnerable cells are exposed to damaging 'hypoxic' changes.

It is not known at what stage in the development of senile dementia cerebral blood flow is reduced. If reduction in flow is secondary to reduced neuronal activity, this implies that metabolic rate is reduced in the nerve cells involved. A reduction in the cerebral metabolic rate results in a reduction in flux through the Krebs cycle and in the concentration of lactate (Thurston et al, 1975). In hypoxia the flux through the Krebs cycle declines, but lactate content is increased. The changes detected in experimental ischaemia may not be entirely relevant to the dementias and related disorders, in which cerebral blood flow is decreased in the absence of morphological evidence of appreciable cerebrovascular disease.

BIOCHEMICAL INDICES OF BRAIN STRUCTURE

As part of the experiment previously described (page 43) temporal lobes from cases of senile dementia and mixed senile and vascular dementia were analysed. Some of the changes detected are summarised in Figure 3.2. A comparison between the controls and cases of organic 'senile-type' dementia suggest that neurones, but not glia, are affected by the disease. The reliable indicators of neuronal cell function and number (i.e. those which are not affected by differences in either agonal state or postmortem handling) include ganglioside NANA concentration and AChE, CNP and β-galactosidase activity. The reduction in these indicators found in cases of organic 'senile-type' dementia suggests that about half of the nerve cells are lost from the temporal lobe. The RNA/DNA ratio is not a reliable index of the relative number of neurones because of possible differences between cases in postmortem handling. DNA content, which is an index of cellularity, correlates with the ratio of β-galactosidase/β-glucuronidase activities, and this reflects the number of neurones relative to glia. Patients with organic 'senile-type' dementia have lower values than normal subjects for both the ratio and the DNA content. This conforms with the view that cell loss occurs in these disorders (Bowen et al, 1977a).

The morphological findings (Fig. 3.2) suggest that, while the relative degree of nerve cell loss was similar in both groups of demented patients, myelin loss was more pronounced in the cases with mixed senile and vascular dementia. These trends parallel the biochemical changes, for the loss of axonal markers is prominent in the vascular cases. In contrast, the loss of markers of nerve cells and Nissl substance and cell shrinkage as judged by the reduction in RNA content are prominent in non-vascular senile dementia. Colon (1973) made cell counts on cases of Alzheimer's disease and concluded that there was a 57 per cent loss of neocortical neurones. This value is in remarkably good agreement with the mean value (57.5 per cent) for the most affected lobes in our study.

If it is assumed that the morphological changes (Fig. 3.2) in cases of dementia reflect on-going neuronal loss, then the reduction in the total number of nerve cells derived from the biochemical data is an estimate of the total neurone loss. Since the estimate of loss is based on age-matched comparisons, the neuronal loss can be considered as *disease-related.* By these criteria in senile dementia, the mean total disease-related loss was 53 per cent. As far as could be established, the duration of the disease in these patients was seven to eight years. Thus, nerve cells appear to have been lost from the lobes at a rate that exceeds the normal ageing rate by perhaps 5 per cent or more per year.

Selective vulnerability of neurones in the 'abiotrophies'

The 'abiotrophies' are a group of neurological diseases of as yet undetermined cause. They include 'senile dementia', Parkinson's disease and Huntington's chorea. In these diseases there is bilateral symmetry of morphological changes in vulnerable regions.

Evidence for changes in the number or state of specific types of neurones in vulnerable regions was obtained by measuring the concentration of neurotransmitters and their biosynthetic enzymes (Bowen and Davison, 1976).

Parkinson's disease

In patients with Parkinson's disease there was a selective reduction in the concentration of dopamine in the substantia nigra which suggests that there is a defect in dopaminergic neurones. In this condition there is a reduction of CAT and GAD activity in the substantia nigra region, but AAD activity is not significantly reduced. The activity of decarboxylase is reduced in parts of the basal ganglia (Bowen et al, 1977b). More recently it has been reported that binding of GABA to receptor sites in the substantia nigra is reduced (Lloyd, Shemin and Hornykiewicz, 1976).

Huntington's chorea

In patients with Huntington's chorea the concentration of GABA in the striatum is reduced, and this suggests that there is a defect of GABAminergic neurones. GAD activity is also selectively reduced in the striatum. Bennett et al (1976) and Enna et al (1976) have recently reported reduction in the same area of muscarinic cholinergic receptor binding, and of the activity of CAT and of angiotensin-converting enzymes.

It seems, therefore, that the biochemical changes first described in these two diseases are not as selective as was originally thought.

Senile dementia

In cases of senile dementia neither AAD nor GAD activity was reduced in the striatum or substantia nigra compared with controls matched for age, agonal state and postmortem handling. GAD activity was markedly reduced in the neocortex (Fig. 3.7a) but this may be related to a combination of terminal bronchopneumonia and reduced cerebral blood flow (see page 52). There was a correlation between CAT activity and 'senile' morphological changes in postmortem samples of brain from cases of senile dementia (Bowen et al, 1976a). The intensity of senile plaque formation was related to the dementia score (Tomlinson and Henderson, 1976). Furthermore, the cholinergic marker was significantly reduced in the neocortex from postmortem cases of senile dementia (Fig. 3.4) and in biopsy specimens from patients with cerebral atrophy of unknown aetiology (Spillane et al, 1977). In the biopsy specimens, which included cases of Alzheimer's disease (Fig. 3.11), the mean GAD activity was unaltered. This is in clear contrast to the postmortem examples (Fig. 3.7a). Thus, the reduction in GAD activity detected postmortem may be due to agonal and blood flow effects. The reduction in CAT has been substantiated by both Perry and her colleagues at Newcastle and by Davies and Maloney in Edinburgh (Anon, 1977).

Aetiology of abiotrophies

Viruses. The characteristic neurofibrillary and granulovacuolar degenerative changes in senile dementia are also found in Guam–Parkinsonism dementia and Guamian amyotrophic lateral sclerosis. A slow virus may be implicated in the latter cases, since increased reverse transcriptase activity has been found in the brain (Viola et al, 1975). Moreover, an infective agent is associated with Jakob–Creutzfeld disease. There is increased concentration of immune complex in the serum from cases of various chronic neurological diseases of unknown aetiology (Oldstone et al, 1976). Preliminary results from this laboratory show no difference in the concentration of circulatory immune complexes between controls and patients with a provisional clinical diagnosis of senile dementia.

Aluminium. Areas of neurofibrillary degeneration (NFD) consist of matted tangles which are apparently either twisted axonal microtubules or possibly pairs of helically wound filaments (Iqbal et al, 1976). An abnormal protein with properties similar to neurofilament protein has been separated at postmortem from tangle-bearing neuronal perikarya. Intracerebral injection of aluminium produces tangles somewhat similar to those found in organic dementia. The metal ion has been detected in increased concentration in the neocortex from patients with senile dementia (Crapper, 1976). This potentially important finding needs to be substantiated.

'*Immunological*'. Senile plaques can be found in the absence of NFD. In the neocortex in senile dementia, plaques are more abundant than NFD. The plaques, which are frequently associated with blood vessels (Bowen and Davison, 1976), contain a 'core' of IgG

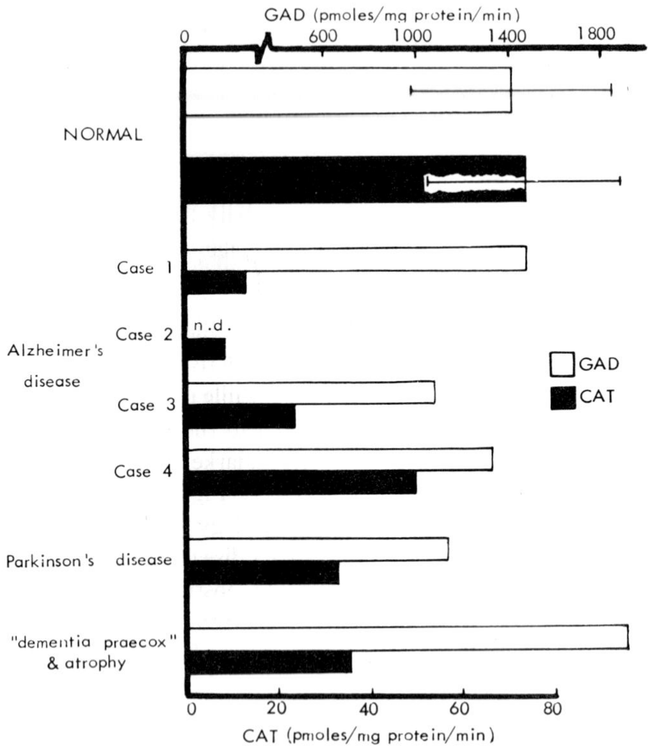

Fig. 3.11 Neurotransmitter-synthesising enzyme activities in cortical specimens removed at surgery (White, 1977; see also Spillane et al 1977); cases 1 and 2 were the more typical of Alzheimer's disease. The case with Parkinson's disease was said to have a sister with presenile dementia. For the normals ($N = 5–7$), the data are the means $\pm$ s.d. GAD = glutamate decarboxylase, CAT = choline acetyltransferase activity

(Ishii and Haga, 1976). This may mean that immunological factors are involved in the pathogenesis of amyloid fibrils in the senile plaques of senile dementia. Immunofluorescent studies have shown an excess of relatively weak antineural reactivity in females with a provisional clinical diagnosis of senile dementia (Mayer, Chughtai and Cape, 1976).

SUMMARY AND CONCLUSIONS

In normal ageing the quality of the nerve cell processes (neuropil) rather than the number of neurones, declines with advancing age, while in organic 'senile-type' dementia there is usually marked loss of neurones. In senile dementia the biochemical changes appear to be more extensive than might be predicted from histopathology. In 'vascular dementia' this is not the case. Thus, in non-vascular senile dementia alteration in the metabolism of neurones may well precede slowly progressive changes in morphology.

There is clinical and neurophysiological evidence of depression of cerebral metabolism in primary neuronal dementia, but cerebral blood flow appears not to be reduced. This implies that an early change in senile dementia may be loss of sensitivity in the central mechanism(s) that regulate the response to changes in the requirement of the neurone for oxygen and nutrients. Research on interaction between the presynaptic cholinergic system, brain metabolism and centrally active peptides might provide clues to the biochemical mechanism(s) leading to brain failure in senile dementia.

REFERENCES

Anon (1977) Cholinergic involvement in senile dementia. *Lancet*, **i**, 408.

Bachelard, H. S. (1976) Biochemistry of coma. In *Biochemistry and Neurological Disease*, ed. Davison, A. N., pp. 228–277. Oxford: Blackwell Scientific Publications.

Barker, J. L. (1976) Peptides: roles in neuronal excitability. *Physiological Reviews*, **56**, 435–448.

Bennett, J. P., Arregui, A. & Snyder, S. H. (1976) Angiotensin II as a possible mammalian central neurotransmitter: synaptic neurochemistry in normal mammalian and Huntington's chorea brain tissue. *Abstracts 6th Annual Meeting of the Society for Neurosciences*, Toronto, p. 775.

Bondareff, W. (1976) Extracellular space in the aging cerebrum. In *Neurobiology of Aging* (*Aging*, Vol. 3), ed. Gershon, S. & Terry, R. D., pp. 167–175. New York: Raven Press.

Bowen, D. M. & Radin, N. S. (1969) Cerebroside galactosidase: a method for determination and a comparison with other lysosomal enzymes in developing rat brain. *Journal of Neurochemistry*, **16**, 501–511.

Bowen, D. M., Smith, C. B. & Davison, A. N. (1973) Molecular changes in senile dementia. *Brain*, **96**, 849–856.

Bowen, D. M. & Davison, A. N. (1974) Macrophages and cathepsin A activity in human brain. *Journal of the Neurological Sciences*, **21**, 227–231.

Bowen, D. M., Davison, A. N. & Ramsey, R. B. (1974) Dynamic role of lipids in the nervous system. In *Biochemistry of Lipids* (MPP International Review of Sciences, Biochemistry Series One), ed. Goodwin, T. W., pp. 141–179. London: Butterworths.

Bowen, D. M. & Davison, A. N. (1976) Biochemistry of brain degeneration. In *Biochemistry and Neurological Disease*, ed. Davison, A. N., pp. 2–51. Oxford: Blackwell Scientific Publications.

Bowen, D. M., Smith, C. B., White, P. & Davison, A. N. (1976a) Neurotransmitter related enzymes and indices of hypoxia in senile dementia and related abiotrophies. *Brain*, **99**, 459–496.

Bowen, D. M., Goodhardt, M. J., Strong, A. J., Smith, C. B., White, P., Branston, N. M., Symon, L. & Davison, A. N. (1976b) Biochemical indices of brain structure, function and 'hypoxia' in cortex from baboons with middle cerebral artery occlusion. *Brain Research*, **117**, 503–507.

Bowen, D. M., Smith, C. B., White, P., Flack, R. H. A., Carrasco, L., Gedye, J. L. & Davison, A. N. (1977a) The chemical pathology of the organic dementias. II. Quantitative estimation of cellular changes in post-mortem brains. *Brain*, **100** 427–453.

Bowen, D. M., Smith, C. B., White, P., Goodhardt, M. J., Spillane, J. A., Flack, R. H. A. & Davison, A. N. (1977b) The chemical pathology of the organic dementias. I. Validity of biochemical measurements in human post-mortem brain specimens. *Brain*, **100** 397–426.

Bradbury, A. F., Smyth, D. G. & Snell, C. R. (1976) C-fragment of lipotropin has a high affinity for brain opiate receptors. *Nature*, **260**, 793–795.

Brody, H. (1976) An examination of cerebral cortex and brainstem aging. In *Neurobiology of Aging* (*Aging*, Vol. 3), ed. Gershon, S. & Terry, R. D., pp. 177–182. New York: Raven Press.

Brown, R. M., Snider, S. R. & Carlsson, A. (1974) Changes in biogenic amine synthesis and turnover induced by hypoxia and/or foot shock stress. II. The central nervous system. *Journal of Neural Transmission*, **35**, 293–305.

Brownstein, M. J., Mroz, E. A., Ikizer, J. S., Palkovits, M. & Leeman, S. E. (1976) Regional distribution of substance-P in the brain of the rat. *Brain Research*, **116**, 299–305.

Byck, R. (1976) Peptide transmitters: a unifying hypothesis for euphoria, respiration, sleep and action of lithium. *Lancet*, **ii**, 72–73.

Clendenon, N. R., Allen, N., Komatsu, T., Liss, L., Gordon, W. A. & Heimberger, K. (1971) Biochemical alterations in the ischaemic-anoxic lesion of rat brain. *Archives of Neurology*, **25**, 432–448.

Colon, E. J. (1973) The cerebral cortex in presenile dementia. *Acta neuropathologica (Berlin)*, **23,** 281–290.

Corsellis, J. A. N. (1962) *Mental Illness and the Ageing Brain,* Maudsley Monograph No. 9. Oxford: Oxford University Press.

Corsellis, J. A. N. (1976) Ageing and the dementias. In *Greenfields Neuropathology*, ed. Blackwood, W. & Corsellis, J. A. N., pp. 796–849. London: Edward Arnold.

Crapper, D. R. (1976) Functional consequences of neurofibrillary degeneration. In *Neurobiology of Aging* (*Aging*, Vol. 3), ed. Gershon, S. & Terry, R. D., pp. 405–432. New York: Raven Press.

Cuello, A. C., Polak, J. M. & Pearse, A. G. E. (1976) Substance-P: a naturally occurring transmitter in human spinal cord. *Lancet*, **ii,** 1054–1056.

Davis, J. & Himwich, W. A. (1975) Neurochemistry of the developing and ageing mammalian brain. In *Neurobiology of Ageing*, ed. Ordy, J. M. & Brizzee, K. R., pp. 329–358. New York: Plenum Press.

Drachman, D. A. & Leavitt, J. (1974) Human memory and the cholinergic system. *Archives of Neurology (Chicago)*, **30,** 113–121.

Duchen, L. W. & Treip, C. S. (1969) Microgliomatosis presenting with dementia and hypopituitarism. *Journal of Pathology*, **98,** 143–146.

Enna, S. J., Bennett, J. P., Bylund, D. B., Snyder, S. H., Bird, E. D. & Iversen, L. L. (1976) Alterations of brain neurotransmitter receptor binding in Huntington's chorea. *Brain Research*, **116,** 531–537.

Fang, H. C. H. (1976) Observations on aging characteristics of cerebral blood vessels, macroscopic and microscopic features. In *Neurobiology of Aging* (*Aging*, Vol. 3), ed. Gershon, S. & Terry, R. D., pp. 155–166. New York: Raven Press.

Finch, C. E. (1976) Endocrine and neural factors of reproductive aging—a speculation. In *Neurobiology of Aging* (*Aging*, Vol. 3), ed. Gershon, S. & Terry, R. D., pp. 335–338. New York: Raven Press.

Gibson, G. E. & Blass, J. P. (1976) Impaired synthesis of acetylcholine in brain accompanying mild hypoxia and hypoglycemia. *Journal of Neurochemistry*, **27,** 31–42.

Goodhardt, M. J., Strong, A. J., Bowen, D. M., White, P., Branston, N. M., Symon, L. & Davison, A. N. (1976) Effect of middle cerebral artery occlusion in baboon on neurotransmitter uptake and neurotransmitter-related biosynthetic enzyme activity. *Biochemical Society Transactions*, **3** 160–163.

Grynbaum, A. & Marks, N. (1976) Characterisation on rat brain catheptic carboxypeptidase (cathepsin A) inactivating angiotensin II. *Journal of Neurochemistry*, **26,** 313–318.

Hachinski, V. C., Iliff, M., Zilkha, E., du Boulay, G. H., McAllister, V. L., Marshall, J., Ross Russell, R. W. & Symon, L. (1975) Cerebral blood flow in dementia. *Archives of Neurology*, **32,** 632–637.

Himwich, C. E. (1973) Neurochemical patterns in the developing and aging brain. In *Development and Aging in the Nervous System*, ed. Rockstein, M., pp. 151–170. New York: Academic Press.

Hughes, J. (1975) Isolation of an endogenous compound from brain with pharmacological properties similar to morphine. *Brain Research*, **88,** 295–308.

Ingvar, D. H. (1976) Functional landscapes of the dominant hemisphere. *Brain Research*, **107,** 181–197.

Ingvar, D. H. & Gustafson, L. (1970) Regional blood flow in organic dementia with early onset. *Acta neurologica scandinavica*, Suppl. 43, **46,** 42–73.

Ingvar, D. H., Risberg, J. & Schwartz Martin, S. (1975) Evidence of sub-normal function of association cortex in pre-senile dementia. *Neurology*, **25,** 964.

Iqbal, K., Grundke-Iqbal, I., Wiśniewski, H. M., Korthals, J. K. & Terry, R. D. (1976) Chemistry of neurofibrous proteins in ageing. In *Neurobiology of Aging* (*Aging*, Vol. 3), ed. Gershon, S. & Terry, R. D., pp. 351–360. New York: Raven Press.

Ishii, T. & Haga, S. (1976) Immuno-electron microscopic localisation of immunoglobulins in amyloid fibrils of senile plaques. *Acta neuropathologica (Berlin)*, **36,** 243–250.

Jablecki, C. & Brimijoin, S. (1975) Axoplasmic transport of choline acetyltransferase activity in mice: effects of age and neurotomy. *Journal of Neurochemistry*, **22,** 583–594.

James, T. C. & Kanungo, M. S. (1976) Alterations in atropine sites of the brain of rats a function of age. *Biochemical and Biophysical Research Communications*, **72,** 170–175.

Katzman, R. (1976) The prevalence and malignancy of Alzheimer's disease. *Archives of Neurology*, **33,** 217–218.

Kuhar, M., Pert, C. & Snyder, S. H. (1973) Regional distribution of opiate receptor binding in monkey and human brain. *Nature*, **245,** 447–450.

Lange, H., Thorner, G., Hopf, A. & Schröder, K. F. (1976) Morphometric studies of the neuropathological changes in choreatic diseases. *Journal of the Neurological Sciences*, **28,** 401–425.

Lloyd, K. G., Shemin, L. & Hornykiewicz, O. (1976) GABA binding in human brain: specific alterations in substantia nigra of Parkinsonian patients. *Abstracts 6th Annual Meeting of the Society for Neurosciences*, Toronto, p. 789.

Lust, W. D., Mrsulja, B. B., Mrsulja, B. J., Passoneau, J. V. & Klatzo, I. (1975) Putative neurotransmitters and cyclic nucleotides in prolonged ischaemia of cerebral cortex. *Brain Research*, **98**, 394–400.

Mayer, P. P., Chughtai, M. A. & Cape, R. D. T. (1976) An immunological approach to dementia in the elderly. *Age and Ageing*, **5**, 164–170.

McGeer, E. G. & McGeer, P. L. (1975) Age changes in the human for some enzymes associated with metabolism of catecholamines, GABA and acetylcholine. In *Neurobiology of Aging*, ed. Ordy, J. M. & Brizzee, K. R., pp. 287–306. New York: Plenum Press.

McGeer, E. G. & McGeer, P. L. (1976a) Neurotransmitter metabolism in ageing brain. In *Neurobiology of Aging* (*Aging*, Vol. 3), ed. Gershon, S. & Terry, R. D., pp. 389–405. New York: Raven Press.

McGeer, P. L. & McGeer, E. G. (1976b) Enzymes associated with the metabolism of catecholamines, acetylcholine and GABA in human controls and patients with Huntington's chorea and Parkinson's disease. *Journal of Neurochemistry*, **26**, 65–76.

Oldstone, M. B. A., Wilson, C. B., Perrin, L. H. & Norris, F. H. (1976) Evidence of immune-complex formation in patients with amyotrophic lateral sclerosis. *Lancet*, **i**, 169–172.

Ordy, J. M., Kaack, B. & Brizzee, K. R. (1975) Life-span neurochemical changes in human and non-human primate brain in clinical, morphologic and neurochemical aspects in the aging central nervous system. In *Aging*, Vol. 1., ed. Brody, H., Harman, D. & Ordy, J. M., pp. 130–190. New York: Raven Press.

Perez, V. J. & Moore, B. W. (1970) Biochemistry of the nervous system in aging. *Interdisciplinary Topics in Gerontology*, **7**, 22–45.

Phillips, M. I. & Felix, D. (1976) Specific angiotensin II receptive neurones in the cat subfornical organ. *Brain Research*, **109**, 531–540.

Poth, M. M., Heath, R. G. & Ward, M. (1975) Angiotensin-converting enzyme in human brain. *Journal of Neurochemistry*, **25**, 83–85.

Robinson, P. S., Nies, A., Davis, J. N., Bunney, W. E., Davis, J. M., Colburn, R. W., Bourne, H. R., Shaw, D. M. & Copper, A. J. (1972) Aging, monoamines and monoamine-oxidase levels. *Lancet*, **i**, 290–291.

Scheibel, M. E. & Scheibel, A. B. (1975) Structural changes in the aging brain. In *Clinical Morphologic and Neurochemical Aspects in the Aging Central Nervous System* (*Aging*, Vol. 1), ed. Brody, A., Harman, D. & Ordy, J. M., pp. 11–38. New York: Raven Press.

Siesjö, B. K. (1977) Physiological aspects of brain energy metabolism. In *Biochemical Correlates of Brain Structure and Function*, ed. Davison, A. N., pp. 175–209. London: Academic Press.

Sokoloff, L. (1976) Circulation and energy metabolism of the brain. In *Basic Neurochemistry*, 2nd edn, ed. Siegel, G. J., Alberg, R. W., Katzman, R. & Agranoff, B. W., pp. 388–412. Boston: Little Brown.

Spillane, J. A., White, P., Goodhardt, M. J., Flack, R. H. A., Bowen, D. M. & Davison, A. N. (1977) Selective vulnerability of neurones in organic dementia. *Nature*, **266**, 558–559.

Tomlinson, B. E. & Henderson, G. (1976) Some quantitative cerebral findings in normal and demented old people. In *Neurobiology of Aging* (*Aging*, Vol. 3), ed. Gershon, S. & Terry, R. D., pp. 183–204. New York: Raven Press.

Thurston, J. H., Hauhart, R. E., Jones, E. M. & Ater, J. L. (1975) Effect of salt and water loading on carbohydrate and energy metabolism and levels of selected amino acids in the brain of young mice. *Journal of Neurochemistry*, **24**, 953–957.

Viola, M. V., Frazier, M., White, L., Brody, J. & Spiegelman, S. (1975). RNA instructed DNA polymerase activity in a cytoplasmic particulate fraction in brains from Guamanian patients. *Journal of Experimental Medicine*, **142**, 483–494.

White, P. (1977) Ph.D. thesis, University of London (in preparation).

White, P., Hiley, C. R., Goodhardt, M. J., Carrasco, L. H., Keet, J. P., Williams, I. E. I. & Bowen, D. M. (1977) Neocortical cholinergic neurones in elderly people. *Lancet*, **i**, 668–670.

Wimersma-Greidanus, T. J. B. van & Wied, de D. (1977) The physiology of the neurohypophysial system and its relation to memory processes. In *Biochemical Correlates of Brain Structure and Function*, ed. Davison, A. N., pp. 215–248. London: Academic Press.

Yamamura, H. I., Kuhar, M. J., Greenberg, D. & Snyder, S. H. (1974) Muscarinic cholinergic receptor binding: regional distribution in monkey brain. *Brain Research*, **66**, 541–546.

Yates, P. O. (1976) Vascular diseases of the central nervous system. In *Greenfield's Neuropathology*, ed. Blackwood, W. & Corsellis, J. A. N., pp. 86–147. London: Edward Arnold.

4. Falls in the elderly—epidemiology, aetiology and management

P. W. Overstall

A hospital serving a catchment area of approximately 210 000 inhabitants, 33 000 of whom are aged 60 years and over might expect an average of 16 beds to be occupied by elderly people admitted because of a fall (Lucht, 1971). However, this is only part of the problem. Very many falls result in no injury, and statistics do not reveal the fear, humiliation and discomfort suffered by elderly people with repeated falls. They may become so fearful of falling that they never venture outside their homes. A pattern of immobility is established, and before long costly support is needed from community services.

Since Sheldon (1960) wrote his now famous paper on the natural history of falls, useful progress has been made in defining the role of cardiac syncope and orthostatic hypotension in falls in the elderly. Although our understanding of the fundamental defect in postural control has advanced very little, there is now an increased awareness that many accidental falls are preventable and some causes of falling remediable.

EPIDEMIOLOGY

The prevalence of falls in the elderly is higher than is generally realised. One of the first studies of a random sample of the elderly population was conducted in Wolverhampton (Sheldon, 1948). Forty-three per cent of women and 21 per cent of men aged 65 and over gave a history of falls. Very similar figures were reported by Exton-Smith (1977) who examined 427 women and 536 men aged 65 and over living in their own homes. He found that in women the proportion who fell increased linearly with age from about 30 per cent in the 65 to 69 age group to just over 50 per cent in those aged 85 or more. For men the proportion who fell increased from 13 per cent in the 65 to 69 age group to 31 per cent in the 80 to 84 age group; thereafter there was a slight decrease in incidence in those aged 85 and over, perhaps representing the survival into extreme old age of exceptionally fit men.

Most of these falls produce no injury. The number who require treatment following a fall in the home is quite small: the annual rate is between 14 and 19/1000 people aged 60 years and over (Lucht, 1971; Waller, 1976). This compares with an annual rate of one-third of the entire elderly population who have falls. Repeated falls are common, especially in those with other diseases. In patients who fell three or more times in a year those with medical illnesses outnumbered the healthy by about three to one (Waller, 1976).

Site of fall

About 70 per cent of falls leading to a femoral neck fracture occur indoors (Clark, 1968; Brocklehurst et al, 1976), usually in the living-room or bedroom. Stairs are an important area of risk. Within institutions most falls are associated with getting in and out of bed, on and off a chair or wheelchair and when using the bathroom (Fine, 1959; Rodstein, 1964). Outdoors, falls occur mainly on the pavement or on the front and back steps of the home.

Time of fall

At home 85 per cent of falls occurred during the day, with a particularly high incidence in the morning and afternoon (Lucht, 1971; Brocklehurst et al, 1976). In hospital most falls occurred at night, usually when the patients were getting out of bed to visit the lavatory. Throughout the 24 h the number of falls was inversely related to the number of staff on duty (Fine, 1959; Manjam and MacKinnon, 1973). In a residential home falls were found to be most frequent at times of maximum activity, in the morning and between 5 and 9 p.m. (Rodstein, 1964). A period of poor light, such as twilight, is a common time for a fall. A minor reduction in visual acuity in persons over the age of 75 is associated with femoral neck fractures (Brocklehurst et al, 1976). Most outdoor falls leading to fracture of the neck of the femur occur during July and August, whilst indoor falls are most frequent in March and April. However, the seasonal variation is not statistically significant (Brocklehurst et al, 1976). Sunday is the commonest day for falls and, indeed, for all types of accident in the home. This probably reflects the increased time spent in the house (Lucht, 1971; Department of Prices and Consumer Protection, 1976).

Social factors

The incidence of falls is highest among widows, widowers and divorcees (Lucht, 1971; Brocklehurst et al, 1976). In patients under the age of 75 years femoral neck fractures are commonest in those living with their children, while in those aged 75 and over the fracture patients live alone.

AETIOLOGY

Falling is not in itself a diagnosis but merely a symptom (Naylor and Rosin, 1970). The tendency to fall may be an indication that the person is no longer able to move within his environment as smoothly and as safely as he did when he was younger; it may be directly due to ill health; or to both factors.

Changes in gait

Most people, as they grow older, are aware that they trip or stumble more frequently. They often blame this on the fact that they no longer pick up their feet as high as they used to. This alteration in gait appears to be a physiological accompaniment of ageing, and differs in the two sexes. Women develop a narrow walking and standing base and walk with more of a waddle, whilst men adopt a flexed posture, a wide walking and standing base and a small-stepped gait (Azar and Lawton, 1964).

Muscular control

Elderly women have less muscular control when they step down from a height than men or young women, and tend to hit the ground more forcefully. Whether this jarring step down is the cause of an occasional spontaneous fracture of the neck of the femur is not clear. In young adults the drop from an unexpected fall must be at least 18 cm to produce a comfortable landing (Melvill Jones and Watt, 1971). Distances shorter than this do not allow sufficient time for the build-up of tension in the leg muscles; a process that is triggered by a central reflex originating in the otoliths, and which one would expect to be slowed with advancing age. A young person who trips is saved from falling by the speed of his postural reflexes, but an elderly person is unable to correct the ensuing disequilibrium.

Postural instability

Postural instability, as measured by an ataxiameter, increases with advancing age, and is more marked at all ages in women than in men (Overstall et al, 1977). Those who fall because of trips sway no more than non-fallers of the same age; while those with increased sway fall because of giddiness, drop attacks, turning the head or after rising from a bed or chair. A distinction may be made between those whose falls are largely due to disease, and those who trip because of a physiological decline in postural control. Gray (1966) and Waller (1976) also found that where a health defect was not the cause most falls were the result of tripping.

Impaired balance in the elderly is due to multiple changes in the neuromuscular system. The literature has been reviewed by Hasselkus (1974), who concluded that although feedback is impaired by changes in joints, muscle spindles and peripheral nerves, it is the slowing in central processes which perceive and integrate proprioceptive signals that is mainly responsible for increased reaction time. This slowing in central processes is largely due to degeneration of the cerebellum and its connections, and sets limits much lower than those set by muscles (Welford, 1962).

ACCIDENTAL FALLS

Trips and accidental falls account for between one-third and one-half of all falls in the elderly (Sheldon, 1960; Clark, 1968; Exton-Smith, 1977; Overstall et al, 1977). However, there is a decline with advancing age in the proportion of falls due to this cause. Thirty-two per cent of men and 37 per cent of women under the age of 75 years attributed their falls to tripping, compared to 28 per cent of men and 22 per cent of women aged 75 years and over. Exton-Smith (1977) considers that this difference is due to the greater mobility of the younger group compared with the incapacity of the older who fall for other reasons, such as giddiness or drop attacks. Brocklehurst et al (1976) confirmed that in patients with femoral neck fractures those who tripped were younger and were more likely to have normal clinical findings on examination of the central nervous system than those who fell for other reasons.

Pathological trips

Frequently falls result from a trip in patients with various pathological gaits. These include the apraxic with retarded initiation of movement of the feet and a tendency to lean backwards due to frontal lobe disease; the hypokinetic–hypertonic with muscle rigidity and slow, short, deliberate steps manifesting extrapyramidal dysfunction; the marche à petits pas typical of the arteriopath; the shuffle of Parkinson's disease and the waddling gait of generalised muscular weakness and arthritis (Barron, 1967). Visual and motor inattention frequently cause trips, but, as Brain (1964) pointed out, the hemiplegic patient rarely falls since considerable concentration is required in order to walk at all.

Mortality

The proportion of patients attending an accident and emergency department following a home accident who are over the age of 65 years is low (Department of Prices and Consumer Protection, 1976). Yet of the 6500 accidental deaths in the home and residential institutions every year (a figure similar to the annual number of deaths on the road), elderly people account for two-thirds. Most are due to falls and some 4000 elderly people die each year in England and Wales from the result of a fall (Alphey and Leach, 1974). Women are affected two to three times as frequently as men. There is a marked seasonal variation, most deaths occurring in winter and fewest in summer. Mortality from accidental falls is highest in Scotland and lowest in the south of England. This is probably due to population differences in height; the average body size declining from south to north of the United Kingdom (Eddy, 1973). The mortality rate is closely related to the frequency of fractures, and larger body size and greater height are associated with less bone loss with age. Osteomalacia contributes to the high incidence of fractures in the elderly (Jenkins et al, 1973) and one would expect to find geographical differences related to average hours of sunshine.

Environmental factors

A detailed study of home accidents among the elderly was made by Gray (1966). Eighty-five per cent of the accidents were falls. Women over the age of 80 with limited mobility were most at risk. The most important causes of falls were ill health, use of defective equipment, and normally harmless objects in situations which created a temporary danger, such as loose mats and steep, dark stairs. Svanström (1975) reported that U-shaped two-flight stairs caused substantially fewer accidents than straight single flights. Three-quarters of falls on stairs occurred when the person was descending. Ten per cent of people blamed their footwear for the fall. The use of the term 'accident', with its pejorative implications of carelessness or thoughtlessness, has been criticised by Waller (1974) who points out that neither the occurrence nor the severity of these events is random. The environment of many old people is frequently hazardous because of trailing wires, loose rugs, missing stair rods, outside lavatories and poor lighting (Agate, 1970). Walking aids and wheelchairs are responsible, in part at least, for some falls, though it is not clear whether the fault lies with the design or with inappropriate use (Waller, 1976). Chairs, beds, carpets and floors account for some of the most expensive accidents in terms of medical costs (Department of Prices and Consumer Protection, 1976). In one series of fractures of the neck of the femur, Clark (1968) estimated that a quarter were clearly preventable and a half possibly preventable by alteration of the environment.

DROP ATTACKS

A drop attack is a sudden fall without warning; consciousness is not lost and there are no neurological sequelae although frequently the patient is unable to rise unless helped.

Age and sex distribution

The condition is almost confined to women. In one series of 40 patients (Stevens and Matthews, 1973) all were women. Overstall et al (1977) found that out of 21 people aged 65 and over who suffered drop attacks, only one was male. With advancing age, however, the number of men affected increases. In men aged 75 and over drop attacks accounted for 7 per cent of falls (Exton-Smith, 1977).

Drop attacks affect at least 3.5 per cent of adult women (Stevens and Matthews, 1973), and are responsible for from 12 to 25 per cent of falls in the elderly (Sheldon 1960; Overstall et al, 1977).

Mechanism of drop attacks

For long it has been considered that drop attacks are due to a temporary reduction in blood flow through vertebral arteries. Of 44 subjects aged 60 and over coming to necropsy with a history of drop attacks 30 had severe atherosclerosis in the vertebrobasilar system. Most also had vertigo and other evidence of vertebrobasilar insufficiency (Kameyama, 1965). Other explanations have been proposed. Epilepsy is a cause of drop attacks in children (Lennox and Lennox, 1960) but no epileptic discharges were seen in electroencephalograms recorded on adults with drop attacks (Stevens and Matthews, 1973). Another hypothesis is that drop attacks occur because an unstable body position is induced by the false interpretation of visual stimulation and is not corrected by postural feedback. In experiments where visual and postural stimulation are set into conflict, women are found to be more 'field dependent' than men: that is they rely greatly on the spatial framework provided by vision. It is possible that the elderly rely more on vision to compensate for a reduced ability to use postural stimulation, and that drop attacks may result from the failure of postural processes to correct an unstable body position induced by reliance on a false visual framework (Over, 1966).

Vertebrobasilar ischaemia, whether or not it is accentuated by cervical spondylosis, may certainly cause drop attacks. This probably accounts for the increasing frequency of drop attacks with advancing age, and for those sudden falls which are preceded by giddiness. Stevens and Matthews (1973) exclude such patients from their series in which the onset of drop attacks was most frequent between the ages of 40 and 59. Of their eight patients with onset before the age of 30, five were pregnant. The falls were frightening and painful but did not have a serious prognosis. Occlusive vascular disease was thought to be an unlikely cause for such brief events which were unaccompanied by other symptoms and which recurred over many years. The explanation might lie in differences between the two sexes at a level more peripheral than the brainstem and possibly related to the mechanism of walking.

Sheldon (1960), noted the loss of tone in the trunk and leg muscles following a drop attack which often persisted for several hours. He postulated that there was a sudden loss of postural alertness through a disturbance of function in the reticular formation. He described how pressure on the soles of the feet against a wall or by the patient being helped to stand, appeared to bring about a recovery of normal tone in the antigravity muscles.

ORTHOSTATIC HYPOTENSION

Orthostatic hypotension is defined as a fall in systolic blood pressure of more than 20 mmHg between the lying and standing position. Between 4 and 6 per cent of falls can be directly related to a change in posture from the lying or sitting to the standing position (Sheldon, 1960; Overstall et al, 1977). The prevalence of orthostatic hypotension is much higher than this. Hypotension is probably also a factor in falls that are blamed on giddiness and loss of balance. Many elderly people are aware of the symptoms and consciously alter their habits to avoid a fall.

Johnson et al (1965) found this condition in 17 per cent of hospital patients aged 70 and over. All the patients with a postural fall in blood pressure had evidence of cerebrovascular disease, and none was taking drugs known to cause orthostatic hypotension. Physiological observations on nine of these patients indicated that the instability of blood pressure probably resulted from a lesion in the central nervous system. At necropsy ischaemic lesions were found at many sites in the brain but not in the spinal cord. Caird, Andrews and Kennedy (1973) showed that in persons aged 65 and over living at home the prevalence of orthostatic hypotension was as high as 24 per cent. A fall of blood pressure of 20 mmHg or more occurred after standing for 1 min in 16 per cent of the 65 to 74 age group and in 30 per cent of those aged 75 years and over, while a postural fall of 30 mmHg or more occurred in 9 per cent of the subjects. Twenty-nine per cent of those whose blood pressure fell by 20 mmHg or more and 22 per cent of those whose blood pressure did not fall had been taking a drug liable to cause orthostatic hypotension. This difference was not statistically significant. There was no sex difference between the groups and there was no association between orthostatic hypotension and organic brain disease or heart disease, but there was a trend towards a greater degree of ill health.

A reduction in blood pressure may be produced by a fall in the circulating blood volume, impairment of circulatory reflexes or disease of the heart. The fall in pressure is accentuated on sitting up or standing, and if the blood supply to the brain is reduced the subject feels giddy or may lose consciousness. Blood volume diminishes during the night which is why symptoms of postural hypotension are common on rising in the morning (Bannister, Ardill and Fentem, 1969). Prolonged bedrest adversely affects orthostatic tolerance (Fareeduddin and Abelmann, 1969). Blood volume may also be reduced in patients with diarrhoea, diabetes mellitus and insipidus, Addison's disease and during treatment with diuretics. The hypotensive effects of myocardial infarction, dysrhythmia and exaggerated circulatory reflexes, such as is seen in carotid sinus syncope, are discussed later.

Impairment of circulatory reflexes

The reflex may be interrupted in the afferent, efferent or central parts of the arc. A central lesion may be in the brainstem or spinal cord (Johnson and Spalding, 1974). Cerebrovascular disease was thought by Johnson et al (1965) to be an important cause of orthostatic hypotension. Following a rapid tilt to 60 degrees, Gross (1970) showed that the postural fall in blood pressure was significantly greater in subjects with cerebrovascular disease than in normal subjects but the duration of the fall was no longer than in controls. The increased fall of pressure in subjects with cerebrovascular disease was not due to increased circulatory reflex latency but was attributed to the effect of gravity on blood contained in a rigid, arteriosclerotic system of vessels.

Idiopathic orthostatic hypotension has been described by many authors. In the syndrome described by Shy and Drager (1960) hypotension presents mainly in middle-aged men and is accompanied by impotence, giddiness, urinary difficulties, fatiguability and loss of sweating. Over several years the autonomic system may fail completely. Olivopontocerebellar atrophy and Parkinsonism may also occur. The orthostatic hypotension results from a defect of reflex vasoconstriction in both resistance and capacity vessels. At necropsy there is marked cell loss at the site of sympathetic preganglionic cell bodies in the intermediolateral columns (Johnson and Spalding, 1974).

Patients with chronic polyneuropathy are also liable to suffer orthostatic hypotension. Of 337 diabetics, 69 had some impairment of circulatory reflexes (Sharpey Schafer and Taylor, 1960). Porphyria and alcoholism may be associated with autonomic disturbances and so may tabes dorsalis when the afferent arc from the baroreceptors is damaged. Patients with chronic loss of circulatory reflexes have only a small drop in blood pressure on standing to which they appear to be well adapted (Barraclough and Sharpey Schafer, 1963). However, they can develop severe orthostatic hypotension if they take drugs which act on central or efferent vasomotor pathways and dilate peripheral veins. In the elderly, in whom the efficiency of circulatory reflexes is commonly impaired, therapeutic doses of many drugs cause symptoms of orthostatic hypotension. These include barbiturates, phenothiazines, benzodiazepines, alcohol, tricyclic antidepressants, monoamine oxidase inhibitors and antihypertensive agents, particularly the adrenergic neurone blockers.

In elderly patients with Parkinson's disease, who exhibit orthostatic hypotension, it is not always clear whether this is due to an age effect, to the disease itself or to drugs used in treatment. Middle-aged Parkinsonian patients with normal baroreceptor reflexes have significant orthostatic hypotension, compared with age-matched controls, which suggests the possibility of a central defect acting above the level of the medulla (Gross, Bannister and Godwin Austen, 1972). L-Dopa can cause a postural fall in blood pressure by altering brain catecholamine concentration, as well as by impairing peripheral baroreceptor reflexes. This effect is reduced when an extracerebral decarboxylase inhibitor is added (Reid et al, 1972).

CARDIAC SYNCOPE

A fall may be caused by any sudden drop in cardiac output from myocardial infarction, pulmonary embolism or a change in cardiac rhythm. The reduction in cerebral blood flow may cause syncope or giddiness without actual loss of consciousness.

Dysrhythmias and conduction defects

Livesley and Atkinson (1974) estimated that 50 per cent of falls observed in 76 elderly patients were a result of unstable cardiac rhythm. Whilst this is certainly too high an estimate, dysrhythmias or atrioventricular block should be considered in those patients who attribute their falls to attacks of giddiness or loss of balance and possibly to those with drop attacks. Giddiness before the fall is only brief. A clear history of loss of consciousness with rapid recovery points to a diagnosis of syncope, especially when there is pallor, absent or very slow pulse and facial flushing on recovery. Between attacks the electrocardiogram was normal in 56 per cent of patients, and in 24 per cent there was a mild dysrhythmia or conduction defect (Van Durme, 1975). The presence of symptoms and dysrhythmia in the same patient does not establish cause and effect unless they occur simultaneously. The diagnosis can often only be made with the help of continuous electrocardiographic monitoring on a portable tape recorder. Van Durme (1975) monitored 95 patients suffering from dizziness or syncope. In 48 per cent the symptoms were accompanied by dysrhythmia, most frequently the sudden onset of supraventricular tachyarrhythmia.

Carotid sinus syncope

Carotid sinus syncope may be suspected if a fall is produced by a sharp turn of the head or by looking up, especially if a tight collar is worn. Ritch (1976) performed the carotid sinus stimulation test on 100 patients admitted to a psychogeriatric unit and found an abnormal cardio-inhibitory response in two patients and a borderline response in 13. The incidence was higher in males, but age alone, arteriosclerosis and coronary artery disease were not predisposing factors.

Sick sinus syndrome

This syndrome occurs commonly in the eighth decade. The characteristic electrocardiogram shows chaotic atrial activity, changing P-wave contours, bradycardia and runs of atrial and nodal tachycardia. The condition may be symptomless, or the changes in cardiac rhythm may cause falls.

Miscellaneous causes

Falls may be due to bradycardia in patients treated with digoxin or beta-blockers. Rarely syncope may occur during micturition, defecation, swallowing and coughing.

GIDDINESS

This is mainly a problem of the very old. Seven per cent of men and 6 per cent of women under the age of 75 attributed their falls to giddiness, compared with 20 per cent of men and 16 per cent of women aged 75 and over (Exton-Smith, 1977). Sheldon (1960) considered that the prevalence of falls associated with giddiness was low because an attack develops slowly and allows time for the person to sit down or hold on. A little over half of the people in his sample who suffered attacks of giddiness had fallen.

There are many causes of giddiness in an elderly person (Dix, 1973), the commonest being vertebrobasilar ischaemia, often precipitated by change in posture or by turning the head. True vertigo, with a sensation of turning, is associated with severe atherosclerosis, especially of the basilar arteries (Kameyama, 1965). Giddiness often appears for the first time during a general illness, in association with anaemia or hypothyroidism, or as a side-effect of drugs, particularly the psychotropics. In the treatment of vertigo cinnarizine is the drug of choice (Dix, 1973).

Cervical spondylosis

Four or five per cent of falls are caused by turning the head (Sheldon, 1960; Overstall et al, 1977). Cervical spondylosis may contribute to falls by producing giddiness. Of 100 patients with cervical spondylosis, 17 presented with giddiness brought on in 10 of those by movements of the head, usually rotation and extension, rarely flexion. Five patients had other symptoms of vertebrobasilar ischaemia, four had attacks of unconsciousness and three had drop attacks (Brain, 1963).

Cervical spondylosis affects nearly everyone over the age of 70. The occurrence of giddiness probably depends on the degree of atheroma of the vertebrobasilar system.

Transient ischaemic attacks

Vertigo and falls are the commonest manifestation of transient ischaemic attacks in the vertebrobasilar territory, but there are usually additional signs of brain stem injury such as diplopia, facial sensory disturbance and dysarthria. Transient ischaemic attacks are considered further in Chapter 6.

PSYCHOLOGICAL ASPECTS OF FALLS

Psychological factors in elderly people who had accidents were examined by Jacobson (1974). Retardation of psychomotor function in depression and organic brain syndrome results in misperception of environmental danger or an inappropriate response. 'Accident-prone' people have distinguishing traits such as impatience, intolerance and irritability which predispose them to injury. Lawton (1967) described the 'indifferent suicide': the elderly person with sensory deprivation and altered thought processes who becomes indifferent to the world and places himself in a hazardous situation beyond his ability to control. Tiredness, restlessness, undue haste and unexplained errors of judgement are frequently present at the time of a fall (Gray, 1966; Svanström, 1974).

Chronic brain syndrome was found in 20 per cent of patients aged 85 and over with fractured neck of femur, and 9 per cent of a control group (Brocklehurst et al, 1976). Dy

(1973) reported that falls in a nursing home occurred twice as frequently in patients with acute and chronic organic brain syndrome as in patients with non-organic brain syndrome.

The elderly are vulnerable to falls following a change of residence, or a bereavement and during periods of emotional upset. Injury following a fall may be accompanied by confusion, depression, lack of confidence and fear of loss of independence. Early mobilisation is required.

Local causes

About 3 per cent of the falls in Sheldon's (1960) study were attributed to weakness of the legs, commonly an unstable joint. Arthritis of degenerative or rheumatoid type was found in 13 per cent of 450 women with a femoral neck fracture (Clark, 1968). Hodkinson (1962) showed that factors significantly related to falls were limitation of hip, knee or dorsolumbar movements, bilateral Parkinsonian leg rigidity and a shuffling, small-paced gait. Idiopathic muscle weakness was found in 12 elderly patients (Serratrice, Roux and Aquaron, 1968), who presented with weakness of the pelvic and shoulder girdles and in most cases, the posterior neck muscles. Electromyograms and muscle biopsies showed patchy myopathic changes. Osteomalacia, hypokalaemia and diabetes should be considered as possible causes of muscle weakness and falls.

DRUGS

The falls of some elderly people are due, in part at least, to drugs. Alcohol contributed to 8 per cent of falls mainly in chronic heavy drinkers (Waller, 1976). An association between falls and the taking of barbiturates or tranquillisers has been reported by Rodstein (1964). In hospital patients falls were most common in the second and third hours following administration of a hypnotic (Manjam and MacKinnon, 1973). Hypoglycaemia may cause falls in patients receiving chlorpropamide (Schen and Benaroya, 1976).

Neurological conditions

Diseases of the central nervous system commonly found among patients who require admission to hospital because of a fall (Naylor and Rosin, 1970; Brocklehurst et al, 1976) include chronic brain syndrome, Parkinson's disease, subacute combined degeneration of the spinal cord, subdural haematoma, tabes dorsalis and communicating hydrocephalus.

Osteomalacia

Osteomalacia should be suspected in patients who complain of falls and difficulty in walking, particularly if they have poor sunlight exposure (Hodkinson et al, 1973), are receiving anticonvulsant drugs or have a history of gastrectomy or renal disease.

Hypothyroidism

Lloyd (1967) described 120 patients with hypothyroidism, 77 per cent of whom complained of unsteadiness in walking and in 30 per cent this was of sufficient severity to have caused several falls.

Premonitory falls

These are falls which precede a sudden and often fatal illness, such as chest infection, cardiovascular accident, diarrhoea, gastrointestinal haemorrhage or cardiac failure (Howell, 1971). Rodstein (1964) found that in 147 consecutive accidents within an institution 25 per cent occurred as a manifestation of the onset of acute disease, often a myocardial infarct or an episode of cerebral ischaemia.

MANAGEMENT OF FALLS

As is usual in the practice of geriatric medicine the approach to management should be multidisciplinary. General practitioners and geriatric visitors identify those patients at risk, while they and the hospital team aim to restore the maximum degree of activity and independence. The patient should be made aware of environmental dangers, and the appropriate authority contacted if structural alterations are required in the home. There is a need to educate architects, interior designers and preretirement groups in the application of safety measures.

Patients with orthostatic hypotension should sleep in a sitting position, or with the head of the bed raised, to avoid the harmful fall of blood volume caused by sleeping flat (Bannister et al, 1969). A programme of gradual mobilisation should be started, and a Buxton tilting chair used for sitting the patient out of bed so that he can be rapidly tilted into the recumbent position if he shows signs of cerebral ischaemia. Elastic stockings alone are usually ineffective but they may be helpful in combination with firm bandaging.

There is no treatment for idiopathic drop attacks, although the patient may be advised on how to regain tone in the legs after a fall by pressing the feet against a solid object. Brain (1964), who believed that epilepsy is sometimes a cause, suggested treatment with sodium phenytoin. Patients with drop attacks related to cervical spondylosis may be given a trial of a cervical collar. This must fit well, hold the spine in slight flexion and be worn day and night, but not for longer than three months (Storey, 1971). There is little evidence that the disease is modified by medical treatment (Nurick, 1975). Operation is indicated in rapidly deteriorating cervical myelopathy irrespective of age (Symon, 1971). Occasionally decompression of the vertebral artery is performed.

While syncope following atrial fibrillation or other supraventricular tachycardias may be prevented by digoxin, cardiac syncope is now looked upon as an indication for pacing (Friedberg, 1971). Mild forms of carotid sinus syncope respond to atropine or propantheline, but severe cases need a permanent pacemaker (Bahl et al, 1971). Caution is needed in the sick sinus syndrome because drugs may induce supraventricular tachycardia in patients with bradycardia and vice versa. Pacing is usually preferred (Radford and Julian, 1974).

AFTER THE FALL IS OVER

Many elderly people find it impossible to get up again after a fall. In about half of Waller's (1976) cases the injured person was alone at the time of the fall. Nearly 10 per cent of patients with recent fracture of the femoral neck lay on the ground for between 1 and 6 h before they were rescued (Brocklehurst et al, 1976). In winter this can cause hypothermia. There is a need for the more widespread use of alarm systems with a pull-cord at ground level that can be reached by a person lying on the floor after a fall.

PROGNOSIS

Many elderly people have repeated falls and appear to come to no harm. Loss of confidence may lead to immobility. Patients who require admission to hospital because of falling have a poor prognosis. Naylor and Rosin (1970) found that only 50 per cent in this group were able to leave hospital. Fifty-four per cent died within 18 months of admission, about twice the mortality found by Brocklehurst and Shergold (1969) in all patients discharged from a geriatric unit.

CONCLUSION

The importance of falls as a cause and as a consequence of ill health in the elderly is now recognised. Although much remains to be discovered of the complex background decline in postural control there are, nevertheless, many opportunities for improving the lot of the elderly person who falls.

REFERENCES

Agate, J. (1970) Accidents to old people. *Community Health*, **2**, 29.

Alphey, R. S. & Leach, S. J. (1974) Accidental death in the home. *Royal Society of Health Journal*, **94**, 97.

Azar, G. J. & Lawton, A. H. (1964) Gait and stepping as factors in the frequent falls of elderly women. *Gerontologist*, **4** (2), 83.

Bahl, O. P., Ferguson, T. B., Oliver, G. C. & Parker, B. M. (1971) Treatment of carotid sinus syncope with demand pacemaker. *Chest*, **59**, 262.

Bannister, R., Ardill, L. & Fentem, P. (1969) An assessment of various methods of treatment of idiopathic orthostatic hypotension. *Quarterly Journal of Medicine*, **38**, 377.

Barraclough, M. A. & Sharpey Schafer, E. P. (1963) Hypotension from absent circulatory reflexes. *Lancet*, **i**, 1121.

Barron, R. E. (1967) Disorders of gait related to the ageing nervous system. *Geriatrics*, **22** (11), 113.

Brain, Lord (1963) Some unsolved problems of cervical spondylosis. *British Medical Journal*, **i**, 771.

Brain, Lord (1964) Cerebrovascular disease as a cause of falls in the elderly. *Gerontologia clinica*, **6**, 167.

Brocklehurst, J. C. & Shergold, M. (1969) Old people leaving hospital. *Gerontologia clinica*, **11**, 115.

Brocklehurst, J. C., Exton-Smith, A. N., Lempert Barber, S. M., Hunt, L. & Palmer, M. (1976) Fracture of the femoral neck. *Report No. 1. to the Department of Health and Social Security*.

Caird, F. I., Andrews, G. R. & Kennedy, R. D. (1973) Effect of posture on blood pressure in the elderly. *British Heart Journal*, **35**, 527.

Clark, A. N. G. (1968) Factors in fracture of the female femur. *Gerontologia clinica*, **10**, 257.

Department of Prices and Consumer Protection (1976) *Collection of Information on Accidents in the Home*. London.

Dix, M. R. (1973) Vertigo. *Practitioner*, **211**, 295.

Dy, A. J. (1973) Falling accidents and organic brain syndrome. *New England Journal of Medicine*, **288**, 1026.

Eddy, T. P. (1973) Deaths from falls and fractures: comparison of mortality in Scotland and the United States with that in England and Wales. *British Journal of Preventive and Social Medicine*, **27**, 247.

Exton-Smith, A. N. (1977) Functional consequences of ageing: clinical manifestations. In *Care of the Elderly: Meeting the Challenge of Dependency*, ed. Exton-Smith, A. N. & Grimley Evans, J. London: Academic Press.

Fareeduddin, K. & Abelmann, W. H. (1969) Impaired orthostatic tolerance after bed rest in patients with myocardial infarction. *New England Journal of Medicine*, **280**, 345.

Fine, W. (1959) An analysis of 277 falls in hospital. *Gerontologia clinica*, **1**, 292.

Friedberg, C. K. (1971) Syncope: pathological physiology: differential diagnosis and treatment. *Modern Concepts of Cardiovascular Disease*, **40**, 55.

Gray, B. (1966) *Home Accidents Among Older People*. London: Royal Society for the Prevention of Accidents.

Gross, M. (1970) The effect of posture on subjects with cerebrovascular disease. *Quarterly Journal of Medicine*, **39**, 485.

Gross, M., Bannister, R. & Godwin Austen, R. (1972) Orthostatic hypotension in Parkinson's disease. *Lancet*, **i**, 174.

Hasselkus, E. R. (1974) Aging and the human nervous system. *American Journal of Occupational Therapy*, **28**, 16.

Hodkinson, H. M. (1962) A study of falls and getting up from the floor in the aged. *Practitioner*, **189**, 207.

Hodkinson, H. M., Stanton, B. R., Round, P. & Morgan, C. (1973) Sunlight, vitamin D and osteomalacia in the elderly, *Lancet*, **i**, 910.

Howell, T. H. (1971) Premonitory falls. *Practitioner*, **206**, 666.

Jacobson, S. B. (1974) Accidents in aged. *New York State Journal of Medicine*, **74**, 2417.

Jenkins, D. H. R., Roberts, J. G., Webster, D. & Williams, H. O. (1973) Osteomalacia in elderly patients with fracture of the femoral neck. *Journal of Bone and Joint Surgery*, **55B**, 575.

Johnson, R. H. & Spalding, J. M. K. (1974) *Disorders of the Autonomic Nervous System*. Oxford: Blackwell Scientific Publications.

Johnson, R. H., Smith, A. C., Spalding, J. M. K. & Wollner, L. (1965) Effect of posture on blood pressure in elderly patients. *Lancet*, **i**, 731.

Kameyama, M. (1965) Vertigo and drop attacks. *Geriatrics*, **20**, 892.

Lawton, A. H. (1967) Accidental injuries to the aged and their psychological impact. *Mayo Clinic Proceedings*, **42**, 685.

Lennox, W. G. & Lennox, M. A. (1960) *Epilepsy and Related Disorders*. London: Churchill.

Livesley, B. & Atkinson, L. (1974) Repeated falls in the elderly. *Modern Geriatrics*, **4** (11), 458.

Lloyd, W. H. (1967) Some clinical features of hyper- and hypothyroidism in the elderly. *Gerontologia clinica*, **9**, 337.

Lucht, U. (1971) A prospective study of accidental falls and resulting injuries in the home among elderly people. *Acta socio-medica scandinavica*, **2**, 105.

Manjam, N. V. B. & MacKinnon, H. H. (1973) Patient, bed and bathroom. *Nova Scotia Medical Bulletin*, **52**, 23.

Melvill Jones, G. & Watt, D. G. D. (1971) Muscular control of landing from unexpected falls in man. *Journal of Physiology*, **219**, 729.

Naylor, R. & Rosin, A. J. (1970) Falling as a cause of admission to a geriatric unit. *Practitioner*, **205**, 327.

Nurick, S. (1975) Cervical spondylosis and spinal cord disease. In *Modern Trends in Neurology*, ed. Williams, D., Vol. 6. London: Butterworths.

Over, R. (1966) Possible visual factors in falls by old people. *Gerontologist*, **6**, 212.

Overstall, P. W., Imms, F. J., Exton-Smith, A. N. & Johnson, A. L. (1977) Falls in the elderly related to postural imbalance. *British Medical Journal*, **i**, 261.

Radford, D. J. & Julian, D. G. (1974) Sick sinus syndrome: experience of a cardiac pacemaker clinic. *British Medical Journal*, **iii**, 504.

Reid, J. L., Calne, D. B., George, C. F. & Vakil, S. D. (1972) The action of L(–)-dopa on baroreflexes in Parkinsonism. *Clinical Science*, **43**, 851.

Ritch, A. E. S. (1976) The significance of carotid sinus hypersensitivity in the elderly. *Gerontologia clinica*, **17**, 146.

Rodstein, M. (1964) Accidents among the aged. *Journal of Chronic Diseases*, **17**, 515.

Schen, R. J. & Benaroya, Y. (1976) Hypoglycaemic coma due to chlorpropamide: observations on twenty-two patients. *Age and Ageing*, **5**, 31.

Serratrice, G., Roux, H. & Aquaron, R. (1968) Proximal muscle weakness in elderly subjects. *Journal of the Neurological Sciences*, **7**, 275.

Sharpey Schafer, E. P. & Taylor, P. J. (1960) Absent circulatory reflexes in diabetic neuritis. *Lancet*, **i**, 559.

Sheldon, J. H. (1948) *The Social Medicine of Old Age*. London: Oxford University Press.

Sheldon, J. H. (1960) On the natural history of falls in old age. *British Medical Journal*, **ii**, 1685.

Shy, G. M. & Drager, G. A. (1960) A neurological syndrome associated with orthostatic hypotension. *Archives of Neurology*, **2**, 511.

Stevens, D. L. & Matthews, W. B. (1973) Cryptogenic drop attacks: an affliction of women. *British Medical Journal*, **i**, 439.

Storey, G. O. (1971) Medical treatment. In *Cervical Spondylosis*, ed. Wilkinson, M. London: Heinemann.

Svanström, L. (1974) Falls on stairs: an epidemiological accident study. *Scandinavian Journal of Social Medicine*, **2**, 113.

Symon, L. (1971) Surgical treatment. In *Cervical Spondylosis*, ed. Wilkinson, M. London: Heinemann.

Van Durme, J. P. (1975) Tachyarrhythmias and transient cerebral ischaemic attacks. *American Heart Journal*, **89**, 538.

Waller, J. A. (1974) Injury in aged. *New York State Journal of Medicine*, **74**, 2200.

Waller, J. A. (1976) Falls among the elderly—human and environmental factors. *Accident Analysis and Prevention* (in press).

Welford, A. T. (1962) On changes of performance with age. *Lancet*, **i**, 335.

5. Bone disorders in old age

P. H. Millard   I. R. Hastie

Bone is composed of living cells and a bone matrix, principally collagen, upon which bone salts are deposited. Throughout life, even after cessation of longitudinal growth, cancellous and cortical bone are constantly being replaced. Changes in the balance between formation and resorption underlie diseases affecting the adult skeleton (Harris and Heaney, 1969).

The quantity of bone present at maturity depends upon sex, race, height, body build, posture, exercise and the supply of calcium, protein and vitamin D during growth and development.

The two major diseases of bone in the elderly are osteoporosis and osteomalacia. The former is defined as too little bone of normal composition; the latter as a failure of calcification of bone tissue with accumulation of uncalcified bone matrix (osteoid). Knowledge of the pattern of development and loss of bone with age, and of vitamin D metabolism, is necessary for the understanding of these conditions.

DEVELOPMENT AND LOSS OF BONE WITH AGE

In both sexes the amount of bone in the body increases until the fourth decade, then declines (Garn, 1970). Methods of measuring bone loss have been reviewed by Dequeker (1975) but only the more commonly used ones will be summarised here.

Dimensional measurements

The most commonly used method is a simple dimensional measurement of a long bone such as a metacarpal. The measurements are shown in Figure 5.1.

Exton-Smith et al (1969a) showed that the measurement ($D^2 - d^2$) had the closest correlation with ash weight in the third proximal phalanx. In order to compensate for differences in skeletal size between individuals and between the sexes they used the formula $(D^2 - d^2)/DL$ where DL is an estimate of body size. In a cross-sectional study they demonstrated a reduction in the measurable amount of bone in the second metacarpal, of 20 per cent in women and 10 per cent in men between the ages of 50 and 80 years. The standard deviation from the mean was approximately the same in each age group from 30 to 80 years (Exton-Smith et al, 1969b).

Relationship to age

Percentile ranking curves developed from the data of Exton-Smith et al (1969b) agreed with the model of bone loss constructed by Newton-John and Morgan (1968). These authors attributed the following characteristics to bone loss: '(1) it begins at about 35 to 45 years in women and about 45 to 65 years in men; (2) the fall in the amount of bone is linear with respect to age; (3) the rate of fall as a percentage of the initial mean value is about 10 per cent in women and possibly less in men; (4) the amount of bone at each age has a normal distribution; and (5) the variation in the amount of bone between individuals remains constant with age (i.e. the standard deviation, which is about 12 per cent of the mean at 30 to 40 years, does not change with age)'.

Exton-Smith et al (1969b) suggested that in women the amount of bone was dependent upon age and the amount present at maturity; in men the relationship to age was less close. After the age of 75, the curve flattened and rose slightly in the late 80s. Since the data were derived from a cross-sectional study, this effect may have been due to differential survival into late old age of subjects with relatively large amounts of bone. Morphological measurements of other bones, and densitometry, demonstrate the same pattern in cross-sectional studies (Dequeker, 1975). The few longitudinal studies which have been done confirm the pattern of loss formulated by Newton-John and Morgan (1968).

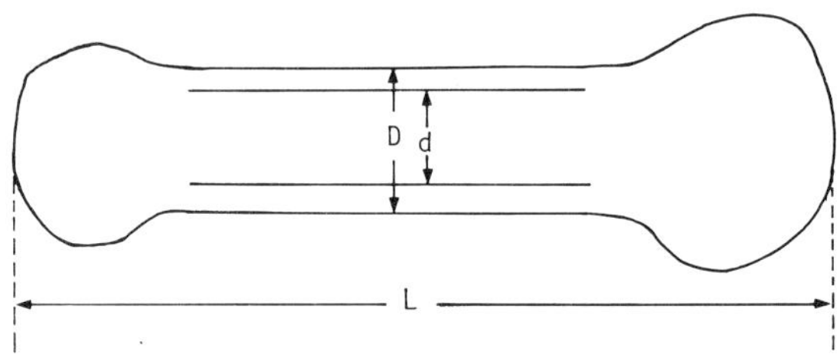

D = External Diameter at the mid-point

d = Internal Diameter at the mid-point

L = Length of Bone

The amount of bone can be expressed as:-

$(D - d)$; $\frac{(D - d)}{D}$; $(D^2 - d^2)$; $\frac{(D^2 - d^2)}{DL}$

Fig. 5.1 Measurements made on longbones (diagrammatic)

Percentile ranking curves indicate whether the amount of bone in a metacarpal is less than expected for the age and sex of the individual, but are of no value in predicting fractures (Adams, Davies and Sweetnam, 1970).

The endosteal envelope phenomenon

Bony material lies outside the bone cells, and remodelling takes place from the surfaces upon which the cells active in remodelling reside. Three surfaces, or 'envelopes', have been defined: the *periosteal*, which lines the outside of all bones; the *endosteal*, which lines the marrow cavities and covers the trabeculae of cancellous bone; and the *intra-cortical*, or Haversian, which lines the Haversian canals.

In the normal adult, most bone cells are inactive. Remodelling is a local phenomenon and proceeds in a uniform sequence. First, a localised subunit of the mesenchyme is activated; then osteoclasts are formed which resorb or remove the subjacent bone surface; after about a month, the osteoclasts disappear and are replaced by osteoblasts formed from mesenchymal precursors which deposit new bone on the previously resorbed surface; and finally, a resting stage is established. The time required to complete this sequence is estimated as from three to four months (Frost, 1973), or from 9 to 15 months (Heaney, 1974). Bone remodelling units are activated by parathormone.

The periosteal surface is predominantly a bone-forming surface, so the external diameter of bones increases with age. The endosteal surface is predominantly a resorbing surface, so the marrow cavity also enlarges with age. Heaney (1974) considers that osteoporosis is determined by selective alteration of the responsiveness of end-organs to parathyroid hormone, but states that as the disturbance in remodelling balance is confined to the endosteal surface, marrow factors may play a part.

Bone collagen

The function of collagen is mainly mechanical. Throughout the body, collagen fibres are stabilised by a system of covalent interchain cross-links. Both intramolecular and intermolecular cross-links increase with age. Bailey, Peach and Fowler (1970) demonstrated that in addition to cross-links, which are stable to weak acids and thermal denaturation, there are also labile cross-links. Fujii, Kuboki and Sasaki (1976) demonstrated that the proportion of soluble collagen in human bone decreased with age from 1.9 per cent of total collagen at three years of age to 0.2 per cent at 18 years and 0.1 per cent at 89 years. Chromatographically the most significant change was that the amount of dihydroxylysinonorleucine (diOH-LNL) decreased markedly with age, while hexitollysines (Hex-lys) and their anhydro-derivatives increased with age.

It is not known whether the increasing cross-linkages which strengthen the bone are eventually deleterious, nor whether the change in solubility of collagen affects bone loss.

Bone salts

Approximately 90 per cent of bone is fibrous collagen protein, the remainder being mainly calcium and phosphorus. A 12-week fetus contains 0.2 g of calcium, a newborn infant contains 80 g, and a mature adult 1100 to 1500 g (Albanese et al, 1975).

A loss of 30 to 50 per cent of bone must occur, by excess of resorption over formation, in order to produce osteoporosis. This means an average loss from the skeleton of 50 mg calcium/day for 20 to 30 years, or of 100 mg calcium/day for 10 to 15 years (Heaney, 1974).

No significant changes occur in bone composition with increasing age.

Dequeker (1975) comments that 'since no significant quantitative differences with age or sex have been reported for the mineral or collagen content of human bone, a concomitant oesteomalacic phenomenon with ageing is not established'. In other words osteomalacia ocurring in old age is a disease and not a general phenomenon of ageing.

Urinary excretion

Dequeker (1972) demonstrated that the urinary excretion of calcium, phosphate and hydroxyproline is decreased in old age. He also showed that there was an inversion of the normal diurnal rhythm, and that in older subjects night excretion of calcium exceeded the day excretion. He considers that the reduced output during the day is probably related to reduced gastrointestinal absorption, or to reduced intake and/or reduced renal excretion.

In this study he demonstrated no marked diurnal rhythm in the excretion of hydroxyproline and considers that the decreased excretion can be explained by a decrease in skeletal mass, and thus of skeletal collagen.

Serum levels

In women under the age of 50 the serum calcium and alkaline phosphatase levels are lower than in men, but in older age groups the sex difference is reversed (Dequeker, 1972).

Young and Nordin (1967) demonstrated in a cross-sectional study that serum calcium, phosphorus and alkaline phosphatase increase in women after the menopause. This rise has been attributed to the lack of oestrogenic protection against parathyroid hormone in women at the menopause.

OSTEOPOROSIS

The definition of osteoporosis as a disorder of too little bone of normal composition has never been seriously challenged (Dent and Watson, 1966). Dequeker (1975) comments that 'if this means too little by the standards for adults in the prime of life, many persons who have no symptoms have osteoporosis simply because physiological changes of ageing have affected their bone'!

There may be two groups of old people with the clinical syndrome of osteoporosis. First, there are those who, having a small bone mass in adult life, have gradually lost sufficient with advancing years to develop clinical osteoporosis. The second group are those with a precipitating cause such as hyperthyroidism, neoplastic disease, scurvy, malabsorption (for example following partial gastrectomy), or spontaneous or iatrogenic Cushing's disease. Prolonged immobilisation can cause bone loss at any age. Hodkinson and Brain (1967) demonstrated significant bone loss in the hemiplegic limb of 10 out of 14 patients, while Goodman (1971) found osteoporosis of the affected side in hemiplegic patients approximately nine weeks after the onset of disability. Osteoporosis was not found in the presence of active motion of the involved extremity.

Clinical features

Osteoporosis classically presents at the time of fracture either of a vertebral body or of a long bone. A collapse fracture of a vertebral body may present with sudden onset of pain in the back, usually following movement. The pain is self-limiting and usually lasts for about six weeks.

Diagnosis

Assessment of osteoporosis in the vertebral column is difficult. X-rays of the spine can be misleading, but points to look for are crush fractures, decreased density of the bones, wedging of the vertebrae, and accentuation of the vertical trabeculation of the vertebral body. There is a close correlation between osteoporosis and backache, but not between backache and x-ray findings. Chronic bone pain almost certainly indicates some other disorder, no matter what the x-ray shows. Even vertebral fractures do not necessarily produce backache.

Gallagher et al (1973) report that 'no absolute morphometric or metabolic difference distinguishes crush fracture patients from the rest of the population, but a limited number of iliac crest biopsies suggests that the fractures occur in patients with a severely reduced amount of trabecular bone'.

TREATMENT OF OSTEOPOROSIS

There is no single definitive treatment of osteoporosis. The basic approach is to look for and treat concomitant conditions.

Therapeutic possibilities

Heaney (1974) comments that there are three ways to shift bone balance towards net formation. One is to decrease the number of remodelling sites. Oestrogens and calcium both do this, but the positive calcium balance effect is short-lived. The second is by interference with the osteoclasts or the bone substrate. Fluoride, calcitonin, pyrophosphate, the diphosphonates, and phosphate do this, but their use is still experimental. The third way is to alter the other parathyroid end-organs, i.e. the kidneys and the intestines, to compensate for the increased sensitivity of bone. This is still largely unexplored territory, but it is known that growth hormone is capable of converting the adult endosteal envelope from a resorbing to a forming surface.

Oestrogens

As yet it has not been conclusively demonstrated that oestrogens are of benefit in preventing bone loss after the normal menopause. Oestrogens are said to be protective against the action of parathormone. Riggs et al (1973) suggested that increased parathyroid function is not a distinguishing feature of most osteoporotic patients and that there may be a partial inhibition of parathormone secretion. Lindsay et al (1976) reported that treatment of 63 oophorectomised women with oestrogens (mestranol) for five years prevented the reduction in bone mineral content observed by densitometry in 57 women treated with a placebo preparation.

Calcium

Therapy with calcium supplementation has had its supporters. Heaney (1974) comments that 'nutritionists argue for a higher calcium intake as effective prophylaxis. It is hard to be against this, but it is also hard to find any convincing epidemiologic relation between calcium intake and osteoporosis risk. It is possible that calcium intake is *the* critical factor for some women, but it is not possible at this time to say which women.' Albanese et al (1975) reported benefit from calcium supplementation in 12 elderly females aged 78 to 86 who had long histories of subnormal dietary calcium levels. They believe that a daily minimum intake of 1 g of calcium throughout life is needed to maintain bone density.

Mobilisation

Mobilisation remains the mainstay of treatment and prevention. The effects of immobilisation and the benefit of exercise were dramatically demonstrated in astronauts. In the early flights Mack and LaChance (1967) demonstrated significant loss of calcium from the bones during a four day flight. The bone lost was regained by 47 days after the flight. Institution of an exercise regime for later flights prevented such bone loss.

VITAMIN D

Vitamin D is the name given to a group of fat-soluble secosteroids, which act by attaching themselves to macromolecules and thus altering their structure. Plant ergosterol is changed by irradiation with ultraviolet light to vitamin D_2 (ergocalciferol). 7-Dehydrocholesterol is similarly changed to vitamin D_3 (cholecalciferol).

In the United Kingdom vitamin D is found in fish oils, margarine (to which it is added in an amount of 2 μg/oz) and in small amounts in eggs and milk. In the United States and Canada milk is also fortified (10 μg/quart).

One milligram of vitamin D_2 or vitamin D_3 is equivalent to 40 000 antirachitic units.

Absorption

Dietary vitamin D is absorbed from the small intestine, mostly in the form of vitamin D_2, in the presence of bile salts which are needed for the formation of micelles. These facilitate transport across the brush border. There is an enterohepatic circulation, vitamin D being secreted in the bile as glucuronides and reabsorbed through the intestinal mucosa.

Most of the circulating vitamin D is in the endogenous D_3 form rather than the exogenous D_2 form, even in the USA where milk is fortified (Haddad and Hahn, 1973).

Vitamin D in the skin

7-Dehydrocholesterol is converted in the skin into vitamin D_3 by the action of ultraviolet light. Whether this occurs on the skin surface (Gaylor and Sault, 1964) or in the malpighian layers (Wheatley and Reinertson, 1958) is debatable. Stamp (1973) considers that only at times of lack of exposure to sunlight is dietary vitamin D_2 required.

NEWER KNOWLEDGE OF VITAMIN D

When vitamin D is given orally there is a delay of 16 to 20 h before calcium absorption from the intestine increases. This is not due solely to delay in intestinal absorption, for even if given intravenously there is a delay of 10 to 12 h (DeLuca, 1975).

25-Hydroxylation

Using radioactively labelled vitamin D_3, Bhattacharyya and DeLuca (1974) found that a process of 25-hydroxylation occurs on the endoplasmic reticulum of the liver cells, converting vitamin D_3 to 25-hydroxycholecalciferol (25-OH-D_3) under the influence of the enzyme vitamin D_3-25-hydroxylase. This is governed, to some degree, by the level of 25-OH-D_3 in the cells. 25-OH-D_3 is released from the liver as it is needed by the body, freeing vitamin D_3-25-hydroxylase to replenish the released 25-OH-D_3. The supply of 25-OH-D_3 for the body remains fairly constant despite the varying intake and skin production of vitamin D_3. Excess 25-OH-D_3 is stored in muscle and adipose tissue. This control prevents toxicity of vitamin D in normal doses, but this safety mechanism may be overridden by an excess of vitamin D (DeLuca, 1975).

25-OH-D_3 is transported in the blood attached to an alpha-globulin. When 25-OH-D_3 is administered, calcium absorption from the gut increases after 4 to 6 h.

1-Hydroxylation

In 1969, by use of tritium-labelled 25-OH-D_3, a hitherto undescribed metabolite of vitamin D was discovered in very small amounts in the cell nuclei of isolated chick intestinal cells, bone cells and kidney cells (Lawson, Wilson and Kodicek, 1969). Fraser and Kodicek (1970) demonstrated that 1-hydroxylation of 25-OH-D_3 occurred in the mitochondria of renal tubular cells. The structure of this compound was defined as 1,25-dihydroxycholecalciferol (1,25-OH_2-D_3) by Lawson et al (1971).

1,25-OH_2-D_3 increases intestinal absorption of calcium within 2 to 3 h of administration, and is believed to be the active metabolite.

Control of synthesis of 1,25-dihydroxycholecalciferol

Until recently it was thought that parathormone acted directly on the bone, intestine and kidney to increase intestinal absorption, mobilisation from bone and renal tubular reabsorption of calcium.

In 1972 Rasmussen et al demonstrated that parathormone is secreted in response to a low serum calcium. It is transported to the renal tubular cells where it activates 1-hydroxylation in association with cyclic AMP and thus converts 25-OH-D_3. A low serum phosphate has also been shown to increase the production of 1,25-OH_2-D_3.

Sites of action of 1,25-dihydroxycholecalciferol

1,25-OH_2-D_3 influences DNA transcription in intestinal cells with the production of a messenger RNA, which produces a protein capable of binding calcium.

In gluten sensitivity, with atrophy of jejunal papillae, there is failure of 1,25-OH_2-D_3 to produce the calcium-binding protein, with a subsequent block to calcium absorption. 1,25-OH_2-D_3 also independently activates phosphorus transport into the intestinal cell.

1,25-OH_2-D_3 is needed for the absorption of calcium from bone to increase the extracellular concentration. In contrast to the action of 1,25-OH_2-D_3 on the gut, this effect also requires parathormone.

1,25-OH_2-D_3 probably acts at the renal tubular level to produce reabsorption of calcium from the tubular lumen; presumably by a mechanism similar to that seen in the intestinal cell (Larkins, MacAuley and MacIntyre, 1974). This increases the calcium concentration in the renal tubular cells, which in turn inhibits 1,25-OH_2-D_3 production, and thus gives a feedback control mechanism.

Regulation of calcium and phosphate concentrations

Hypocalcaemia is recognised by the parathyroid glands which in response secrete parathormone. In the kidney, parathormone facilitates the reabsorption of calcium and stimulates the release of 1,25-OH_2-D_3 which acts alone to increase calcium absorption from the small intestine and together with parathormone to mobilise calcium from bone, thus causing a rise in serum calcium. When serum calcium has reached its normal level the stimulus to parathormone secretion is cut off and the process is stopped.

1,25-OH_2-D_3 also stimulates phosphate absorption from the gut and from bone. In hypocalcaemia, this rise is counteracted by the release of parathormone, producing a phosphate diuresis and thus maintaining a steady phosphate level.

In hypercalcaemia the processes are reversed, with reduced absorption of calcium from the small intestine and reduced mobilisation from bone (DeLuca, 1975).

Calcitonin is secreted from parafollicular 'C' cells in the thyroid glands in response to a raised serum calcium, and restores the level to normal. Calcitonin produces its effect by an action on the bone cells, osteoclasts, osteocytes and osteoblasts (Goodman and Gilman, 1975).

Other metabolites of vitamin D

24,25-dihydroxycholecalciferol (24,25-OH_2-D_3) is synthesised in the kidney in inverse quantities to 1,25-OH_2-D_3. To be metabolically active it is metabolised to 1,24,25-trihydroxycholecalciferol (1,24,25-OH_3-D_3) (Holick et al, 1973), which may be the metabolite used under normal circumstances, but at times of stress, such as dietary deficiency, then 1,25-OH_2-D_3 is needed (DeLuca, 1975). Little is known about the metabolite

25,26-dihydroxycholecalciferol (25,26-OH_2-D_3), but it does increase calcium absorption from the small intestine (Suda et al, 1970).

In summary, the present stage of knowledge of vitamin D metabolism is:

Dietary cholesterol, having been converted to 7-dehydrocholesterol, is further converted in the skin by ultraviolet irradiation into vitamin D_3. Vitamin D_3 is transported to the liver where it is metabolised by mitochondrial enzymes to 25-OH-D_3. There is an enterohepatic circulation, and diseases of the biliary tract and malabsorption states interfere with this process. Excess 25-OH-D_3 is stored in the muscles and adipose tissues. At times of need for calcium, parathormone is secreted. This activates 1-hydroxylation in the renal tubular cells and 25-OH-D_3 is converted into 1,25-OH_2-D_3. 1,25-OH_2-D_3 acts alone to increase intestinal absorption, and possibly renal tubular reabsorption, of calcium, and together with parathormone it mobilises calcium from the bone. This then increases serum calcium which inhibits the excretion of parathormone. Renal tubular loss affects the process of 1-hydroxylation.

These metabolic pathways are similar to those of a hormone. There is a precursor (25-OH-D_3) which is transported to an endocrine organ (the kidney) from where a metabolically active substance (1,25-OH_2-D_3) is secreted which acts on an end organ (intestine and bone). Other metabolites have been identified but their role is not yet clear.

In the absence of skin exposure to ultraviolet light, plant ergosterol, converted into ergocalciferol, follows the same pathway of metabolism in the ergo-form and can be used to stimulate calcium absorption.

OSTEOMALACIA

Lack of vitamin D in the elderly is responsible for the clinical syndrome of osteomalacia.

Clinical features

Symptoms include loss of height, difficulty in walking, especially climbing stairs, and constant low-back pain. Signs are of generalised bone tenderness and a waddling gait associated with a proximal myopathy. The presence of Looser's zones on x-ray over the lateral border of the scapula, first rib, greater trochanter or pubic rami are pathognomonic. Serum biochemistry may show a low or normal calcium, a low phosphorus and raised alkaline phosphatase, but all of these may be normal. Sharland (1975) demonstrated the clinical value of serum alkaline phosphatase iso-enzyme studies in the elderly, but this technique is not widely available.

Iliac crest bone biopsy demonstrates widening of the osteoid seams.

The incidence has been put as high as 4 per cent of admissions to geriatric units (Anderson et al, 1966). Aaron et al (1974) found some evidence of osteomalacia in 20 to 30 per cent of women and about 40 per cent of men with fractures of the proximal femur.

CAUSES OF OSTEOMALACIA

Lack of exposure to sunlight

Haddad and Hahn (1973) demonstrated that most of the vitamin D in the circulation is in the endogenous form (cholecalciferol, vitamin D_3), and therefore suggested that the action of ultraviolet light on the skin was the main source of vitamin D production in the body.

Elderly people tend to expose only their hands and faces to sunlight. The presence of cataracts may necessitate the wearing of wide-brimmed hats and thus reduce sunlight exposure to the face. Atmospheric pollution also cuts down ultraviolet irradiation. The housebound elderly are particularly at risk, since window-glass absorbs ultraviolet irradiation. A vicious circle is set up, with lack of exposure to the sun causing deficient vitamin D production, development of back pain and a myopathic gait which makes getting out of chairs and climbing stairs increasingly difficult. Osteomalacia should be suspected in all housebound people.

In a group of long-stay hospital patients Corless et al (1975) found low levels of plasma 25-OH-D_3.

Dietary vitamin D

The elderly have reduced vitamin D intake (Exton-Smith and Stanton, 1965). Hodkinson et al (1973) found no correlation between vitamin D intake and biochemical indices or proven osteomalacia. Sunlight exposure correlated well with levels of calcium and phosphate, but not of alkaline phosphatase.

Dunnigan and Smith (1965) and Holmes et al (1973) showed an increased incidence of rickets and osteomalacia in the Asian communities of the United Kingdom. This may be associated with the eating of chapattis, but could be due to the relative lack of exposure to sunlight (Gupta, Round and Stamp, 1974).

Liver disease

Vitamin D is fat-soluble and needs bile salts for its absorption. Chronic liver disease can lead to bone disease because of a defect in 25-hydroxylation or interference with the enterohepatic circulation.

Anticonvulsant therapy

Dent et al (1970) suggested that drug-mediated enzyme induction in the liver might be the reason why epileptic patients on therapy with anticonvulsant drugs develop osteomalacia. Stamp et al (1972) considered that this was due to the development of inactive metabolites of vitamin D_3. Maclaren and Lifshitz (1973) demonstrated that the reason may be a block in the hepatic conversion of cholecalciferol to 25-OH-D_3.

Patients with epilepsy who remain on anticonvulsant treatment despite symptoms of osteomalacia have been treated with vitamin D in doses of 4000 units/day. 25-OH-D_3 may be used to treat these cases in doses of 10 μg/day (500 units), but it is not yet commercially available.

The problem of induction of osteomalacia should be considered in all patients on long-term anticonvulsant therapy or barbiturates.

Malabsorption

Any cause of malabsorption in the elderly may lead to the development of osteomalacia because of the enterohepatic circulation of vitamin D and its fat solubility.

Renal disease

The renal tubule is the site of 1-hydroxylation of 25-OH-D_3 to 1,25-OH_2-D_3. This is an explanation for the early occurrence of bone disease in disorders affecting the renal tubules rather than the glomeruli.

PREVENTION AND TREATMENT OF OSTEOMALACIA

Exposure to ultraviolet light encourages vitamin D formation. Supplementation of dietary intake by switching from butter to margarine, which is fortified, may be sufficient.

Treatment with vitamin D, 1.25 mg daily, is necessary in the frank case of osteomalacia. Prolonged usage at this dosage can lead to hypercalcaemia. Bone pain and tenderness usually become worse about two days after starting treatment, but tend to improve after one week. Maintenance therapy should be titrated according to the clinical response to treatment.

The newer metabolites of vitamin D are not yet available for general use. 25-OH-D_3 may be marketed first. 1-α-Hydroxyvitamin-D_3 is chemically very similar to 1,25-OH_2-D_3 but, although cheaper to produce, is only half as effective.

These new analogues, with their shorter half-lives, provide better control and therefore produce less toxicity than vitamin D.

FRACTURES IN THE ELDERLY

The incidence of fractures in persons over 35 years of age has been investigated by a Medical Research Council Working Party (Knowelden, Buhr and Dunbar, 1964). This study documented the dramatic increase in fractures with age, more marked in women than men. For example, fractures of the neck of femur are rare below the age of 60 but thereafter the incidence doubles every five years in women and every seven years in men.

Gallannaugh, Martin and Millard (1976) found a higher incidence of fractures of the neck of femur in a regional survey than was reported in the MRC study, especially in the over 80s. The mortality rate increased with age and was higher in males than females.

The increase with age may be due both to a change in the pattern of falling and to an increase in the liability of the bone to fracture with age because of osteoporosis or osteomalacia. The increasing understanding of the mechanisms underlying the development of osteoporosis and osteomalacia may eventually demonstrate methods to reduce the incidence of fractures in the elderly.

REFERENCES

Aaron, J. E., Gallagher, J. C., Anderson, J., Stasiak, L., Longton, E. B., Nordin, B. E. C. & Nicholson, M. (1974) Frequency of osteomalacia and osteoporosis in fractures of the proximal femur. *Lancet*, **i**, 229–233.

Adams, P., Davies, G. T. & Sweetnam, P. (1970) Osteoporosis and the effects of ageing on bone mass in elderly men and women. *Quarterly Journal of Medicine*, **39**, 601–615.

Albanese, A. A., Edelson, A. H., Lorenze, E. J., Woodhill, M. L. & Wein, E. H. (1975) Problems of bone health in elderly. Ten-year study. *New York State Journal of Medicine*, **75**, 326–336.

Anderson, I., Campbell, A. E. R., Dunn, A. & Runciman, J. B. M. (1966) Osteomalacia in elderly women. *Scottish Medical Journal*, **11**, 429–435.

Bailey, A. J., Peach, C. M. & Fowler, L. J. (1970) Chemistry of the collagen cross-links. Isolation and characterisation of two intermediate intermolecular cross-links in collagen. *Biochemical Journal*, **117**, 819–831.

Bhattacharyya, M. H. & DeLuca, H. F. (1974) Subcellular location of rat liver calciferol-25-hydroxylase. *Archives of Biochemistry and Biophysics*, **160**, 58–62.

Corless, D., Beer, M., Boucher, B. J., Gupta, S. P. & Cohen, R. D. (1975) Vitamin-D status in long-stay geriatric patients. *Lancet*, **i**, 1404–1406.

DeLuca, H. F. (1975) Vitamin D today. *Disease-a-month*, March.

Dent, C. E. & Watson, L. (1966) Osteoporosis. *Postgraduate Medical Journal*, **42**, 583–608.

Dent, C. E., Richens, A., Rowe, D. J. F. & Stamp, T. C. B. (1970) Osteomalacia with long-term anticonvulsant therapy in epilepsy. *British Medical Journal*, **iv**, 69–72.

Dequeker, J. (1972) *Bone Loss in Normal and Pathological Conditions*. Leuven: Leuven University Press.

Dequeker, J. (1975) Bone and ageing. *Annals of Rheumatic Diseases*, **34**, 100–115.

Dunnigan, M. G. & Smith, C. M. (1965) The aetiology of late rickets in Pakistani children in Glasgow. Report of a diet survey. *Scottish Medical Journal*, **10**, 1–9.

Exton-Smith, A. N. & Stanton, B. R. (1965) *Report of an Investigation into the Dietary of Elderly Women Living Alone*, p. 23. London: King Edward's Hospital Fund for London.

Exton-Smith, A. N., Millard, P. H., Payne, P. R. & Wheeler, E. F. (1969a) Method for measuring quantity of bone. *Lancet*, **ii**, 1153–1154.

Exton-Smith, A. N., Millard, P. H., Payne, P. R. & Wheeler, E. F. (1969b) Pattern of development and loss of bone with age. *Lancet*, **ii**, 1154–1157.

Fraser, D. R. & Kodicek, E. (1970) Unique biosynthesis by kidney of a biologically active vitamin D metabolite. *Nature*, **228**, 764–766.

Frost, H. M. (1973) The spinal osteoporoses. Mechanisms of pathogenesis and pathophysiology. *Clinics in Endocrinology and Metabolism*, **2**, 257–275.

Fujii, K., Kuboki, Y. & Sasaki, S. (1976) Ageing of human bone and articular cartilage collagen. Changes in the reducible cross-links and their precursors. *Gerontology*, **22**, 363–370.

Gallagher, J. C., Aaron, J., Horsman, A., Marshall, D. H., Wilkinson, R. & Nordin, B. E. C. (1973) The crush fracture syndrome in postmenopausal women. *Clinics in Endocrinology and Metabolism*, **2**, 293–315.

Gallannaugh, S. C., Martin, A. & Millard, P. H. (1976) Regional study of femoral neck fractures. *British Medical Journal*, **ii**, 1496–7.

Garn, S. M. (1970) *The Earlier Gain and the Later Loss of Cortical Bone. In Nutritional Perspective*, p. 34. Springfield: Charles C. Thomas.

Gaylor, J. L. & Sault, F. M. (1964) Localisation and biosynthesis of 7-dehydrocholesterol in rat skin. *Journal of Lipid Research*, **5**, 422–431.

Goodman, C. R. (1971) Osteoporosis as early complication of hemiplegia. *New York State Journal of Medicine*, **71**, 1943–1945.

Goodman, L. S. & Gilman, A. (1975) *The Pharmaceutical Basis of Therapeutics*, 5th edn, pp. 1540-1543. New York: Macmillan Publishing Co. Inc.

Gupta, M. M., Round, J. M. & Stamp, T. C. B. (1974) Spontaneous cure of vitamin-D deficiency in Asians during summer in Britain. *Lancet*, **i**, 586–588.

Haddad, J. G. & Hahn, T. J. (1973) Natural and synthetic sources of circulating 25-hydroxyvitamin D in man. *Nature*, **244**, 515–517.

Harris, W. H. & Heaney, R. P. (1969) Skeletal renewal and metabolic bone disease. *New England Journal of Medicine*, **280**, 193–202, 253–259.

Heaney, R. P. (1974) Pathophysiology of osteoporosis: implications for treatment. *Texas Medicine*, **70**, 37–45.

Hodkinson, H. M. & Brain, A. T. (1967) Unilateral osteoporosis in longstanding hemiplegia in the elderly. *Journal of the American Geriatrics Society*, **15**, 59–64.

Hodkinson, H. M., Stanton, B. R., Round, P. & Morgan, C. (1973) Sunlight, vitamin D, and osteomalacia in the elderly. *Lancet*, **i**, 910–912.

Holick, M. F., Kleiner-Bossaller, A., Schnoes, H. K., Kasten, P. M., Boyle, I. T. & DeLuca, H. F. (1973) 1,24,25-Trihydroxyvitamin D_3. A metabolite of vitamin D_3 effective on intestine. *Journal of Biological Chemistry*, **248**, 6691–6696'

Holmes, A. M., Enoch, B. A., Taylor, J. L. & Jones, M. E. (1973) Occult rickets and osteomalacia amongst the Asian immigrant population. *Quarterly Journal of Medicine*, **42**, 125–149.

Knowelden, J., Buhr, A. J. & Dunbar, O. (1964) Incidence of fractures in persons over 35 years of age. A report to the MRC working party on fractures in the elderly. *British Journal of Preventive and Social Medicine*, **18**, 130–141.

Larkins, R. G., MacAuley, S. J. & MacIntyre, I. (1974) Feedback control of vitamin D metabolism by a nuclear action of 1,25-dihydroxycholecalciferol on the kidney. *Nature*, **252**, 412–414.

Lawson, D. E. M., Wilson, P. W. & Kodicek, E. (1969) Metabolism of vitamin D. A new cholecalciferol metabolite, involving loss of hydrogen at C-1, in chick intestinal nuclei. *Biochemical Journal*, **115**, 269–277.

Lawson, D. E. M., Fraser, D. R., Kodicek, E., Morris, H. R. & Williams, D. H. (1971) Identification of 1,25-dihydroxycholecalciferol, a new kidney hormone controlling calcium metabolism. *Nature*, **230**, 228–230.

Lindsay, R., Hart, D. M., Aitken, J. M., MacDonald, E. B., Anderson, J. B. & Clarke, A. C. (1976) Long-term prevention of postmenopausal osteoporosis by oestrogen. *Lancet*, **i**, 1038–1041.

Mack, P. B. & LaChance, P. L. (1967) Effects of recumbency and space flight on bone density. *American Journal of Clinical Nutrition*, **20**, 1194–1205.

Maclaren, N. & Lifshitz, F. (1973) Vitamin D-dependency rickets in institutionalised, mentally retarded children on long-term anticonvulsant therapy. II. The response to 25-hydroxycholecalciferol and to vitamin D_2. *Pediatric Research*, **7**, 914–922.

Newton-John, H. F. & Morgan, D. B. (1968) Osteoporosis: disease or senescence? *Lancet*, **i**, 232–233.

Rasmussen, H., Wong, M., Bikle, D. & Goodman, D. B. P. (1972) Hormonal control of the renal conversion of 25-hydroxycholecalciferol to 1,25-dihydroxycholecalciferol. *Journal of Clinical Investigation*, **51**, 2502–2504.

Riggs, B. L., Arnaud, C. D., Jowsey, J., Goldsmith, R. S. & Kelly, P. J. (1973) Parathyroid function in primary osteoporosis. *Journal of Clinical Investigation*, **52**, 181–184.

Sharland, D. E. (1975) Clinical value of serum alkaline phosphatase isoenzyme estimations in the elderly. *Age and Ageing*, **4**, 1–7.

Stamp, T. C. B. (1973) Vitamin D metabolism. Recent advances. *Archives of Disease in Childhood*, **48**, 2–7.

Stamp, T. C. B., Round, J. M., Rowe, D. J. F. & Haddad, J. G. (1972) Plasma levels and therapeutic effect of 25-hydroxycholecalciferol in epileptic patients taking anticonvulsant drugs. *British Medical Journal*, **iv**, 9–12.

Suda, T., DeLuca, H. F., Schnoes, H. K., Tanaka, Y. & Holick, M. F. (1970) 25,26-Dihydroxycholecalciferol, a metabolite of vitamin D_3 with intestinal calcium transport activity. *Biochemistry*, **9**, 4776–4780.

Wheatley, V. R. & Reinertson, R. P. (1958) The presence of vitamin D precursors in human epidermis. *Journal of Investigative Dermatology*, **31**, 51–54.

Young, M. M. & Nordin, B. E. C. (1967) Effects of natural and artificial menopause on plasma and urinary calcium and phosphorus. *Lancet*, **ii**, 118–120.

6. Disturbances of autonomic regulation

A. N. Exton-Smith

Many of the phenomena of ageing can be attributed to progressive loss of homoeostatic capacity. A steady decline in physiological function is reflected in reduction in adaptability and increase in susceptibility to environmental stress. As the years pass there is slow erosion of the capacity for adaptation to the strains imposed by the external environment.

In this chapter the effects of impairment of function of the autonomic nervous system will be discussed with particular reference to the control of blood pressure and thermoregulation. Change in body posture from the lying to the upright position or exposure to low environmental temperature more readily produce orthostatic hypotension or hypothermia in old than in younger individuals, as a consequence of physiological impairment of autonomic function in old age. When in addition there is a pathological process involving the autonomic nervous system the clinical manifestations are even more marked and can be more readily provoked.

PHYSIOLOGY AND PHARMACOLOGY OF AUTONOMIC CONTROL

The chemical transmitters in the nervous system include acetylcholine, 5-hydroxytryptamine (5HT), dopamine, and the catecholamines, adrenaline (epinephrine) and noradrenaline (norepinephrine). They are not only concerned with neurotransmission within the central nervous system but they also play an important role in the control of autonomic function.

The principal transmitter at the autonomic ganglia is acetylcholine and its action at this site is not paralysed by atropine. Ganglion-blocking agents such as hexamethonium and mecamylamine are believed to act by competing for acetylcholine and preventing it reaching the receptor. Since the parasympathetic ganglia are also cholinergic the bulbosacral outflow is affected by ganglion-blocking drugs. Acetylcholine is the neurotransmitter at the postganglionic nerve endings of the parasympathetic system; at some sympathetic nerve endings, namely, the sudomotor fibres supplying the eccrine glands which form the majority of the sweat glands; and at some vasodilator fibres to the muscles. Atropine paralyses these actions of acetylcholine. Noradrenaline is the principal transmitter substance for the postganglionic sympathetic nervous system. The adrenoreceptors are of two types which are differentiated on the basis of the relative potencies of adrenergic agents, for example, noradrenaline, adrenaline and isoprenaline. Noradrenaline predominantly stimulates the α-receptors; its effects include vasoconstriction, intestinal relaxation, and pupillary dilation. These actions are blocked by phentolamine and phenoxybenzamine. The β-receptors are stimulated by isoprenaline, and both α- and β-receptors are stimulated by adrenaline. The main effects of β-receptor stimulation are vasodilatation, especially in the muscles, increase in the rate and force of cardiac contraction with a tendency to develop arrhythmias and bronchial dilatation. The blocking agents include propranalol and practalol.

Recently dopamine has been found in significant amounts not only in the central nervous system but also in the autonomic ganglia and nerves. Dopamine receptors have been described in the peripheral autonomic nervous system. They are stimulated by dopaminergic agonists, including apomorphine and bromocriptine, and they are blocked by dopaminergic antagonists such as phenothiazines and metoclopramide, and to a less extent by adrenoreceptor antagonists (Thorner, 1975). Thus dopamine has functions in regulating sympathetic (and probably parasympathetic) activities in the ganglia and probably also at adrenergic nerve endings. The specific dopamine effects can be demonstrated by first blocking the α- and β-receptors and then administering dopamine. The latter can then be blocked by dopamine antagonists. In Parkinsonism, deficiency of dopamine may lead to unopposed action of acetylcholine, with peripheral manifestations such as greasy skin, excessive sweating and vasomotor instability. These effects are reversed by the administration of L-dopa (the precursor of dopamine) or dopamine-receptor stimulating drugs, such as bromocriptine. Overdosage with bromocriptine produces a syndrome of nausea and vomiting, severe hypotension with a postural component, and involuntary repetitive yawning.

Neurochemical changes with age

There have been few studies of the effect of ageing on neurotransmission. Frolkis and his colleagues (1973) of the Institute of Gerontology in Kiev investigated acetylcholine metabolism in adult and old rats, rabbits and cats at sites of acetylcholine action, namely, the vascular receptors, the nervous centres specially in the hypothalamic area, the autonomic ganglia and the cholinergic peripheral effector system. The biosynthesis and hydrolysis of acetylcholine were found to decrease with increasing age. There was a decrease in choline acetyl-transferase and cholinesterase activity, but an increase in the sensitivity of cholinoreceptor protein to acetylcholine. Repeated stimulation led to weakening of the reactions and rapid exhaustion of the reflexes from the vascular chemoreceptor sites. Since the number of receptors is diminished in old age the overall effect was reduction in the functional efficiency of the autonomic reflex arcs.

Bowen and his co-workers (1974) measured decarboxylase activities immediately after death in the brains of patients with varying degrees of dementia. The activity of L-dopa decarboxylase (DOPAD) and of glutamic acid decarboxylase (GAD), enzymes involved in the synthesis of the neurotransmitters dopamine and γ-aminobutyric acid, decreased with age, more markedly in patients suffering from dementia. One explanation for the reduction in GAD and DOPAD activity is that widespread fall-out of dopamin-ergic and GABA-ergic neurons, beginning at the synapse, occurs prematurely in senile dementia. Studies of thermoregulatory function in old people (see page 86) indicate that there may be involvement of the autonomic nervous system in dementia.

PHYSIOLOGICAL CHANGES WITH AGE

Examination of the elderly population living at home indicates that impairment of autonomic function is common in old age.

Cardiovascular reflexes

Caird and his colleagues (1973) found that the incidence of postural hypotension increased with age. A fall of 20 mmHg or more in systolic pressure was observed in 16 per cent of subjects aged 65 to 74 years and in 30 per cent of those aged 75 and over. They believed that autonomic dysfunction was the underlying cause and that this commonly interacted with other factors (see page 90). Gross (1970) also found that impairment of circulatory reflexes, manifested by abnormality of the blood pressure response to Valsalva's manoeuvre, increased in frequency with advancing age. Strandell (1964) observed that the mean increase in heart rate on standing in middle-aged and elderly subjects, was 10 to 15 beats/min compared with approximately 20 beats/min in young adults. Bristow and his colleagues (1969), by recording the reflex bradycardia produced by the rise in pressure following intravenous injection of phenylephrine (25–100 μg) found a diminished baroreflex sensitivity with increasing age. They suggested that this might be due to decreased distensibility with increasing age of the arterial wall at the baroreflex site.

Thermoregulation

Thermoregulatory function has also been investigated in the elderly population. Fox and his colleagues (1973a) measured body temperature in a random sample of 1020 people aged 65 and over living at home in Great Britain during the first three months of 1972. Deep body temperature, as measured by urine temperature, was significantly correlated with advancing age. In 10 per cent of subjects the deep body temperature was less than 35.5°C. The core-peripheral temperature gradient in this 'low' temperature group was significantly less than in the group where deep body temperatures were 36.0°C and above (see page 92).

Foster and his colleagues (1976) found a diminution of sweat responses to thermal stimulation and to the intradermal injection of acetylcholine, more marked in the limbs than in the trunk, with increasing age. Of subjects aged 60 and over one half showed a diminished or absent response.

These observations on decline in function in the autonomic nervous system were made in cross-sectional studies. There have been few longitudinal studies of autonomic function. Collins and his co-workers (1977) investigated the changes in thermoregulatory function with age by measurements repeated after an interval of four years on the surviving participants of an intensive study in Camden in 1972. These serial measurements revealed a decline in function in the autonomic nervous system in each individual. A higher proportion of subjects had low resting peripheral blood flow, abnormal vascular response to cold and postural hypotension. There was also an age-related increase in the temperature required for the onset of sweating.

PATHOLOGICAL CHANGES

The autonomic nervous system may be involved in a number of pathological processes. The most widespread involvement occurs in the Shy–Drager syndrome. Although this is a rare disease it will be described first, since all the manifestations of autonomic failure are to be found in the clinical picture.

Shy–Drager syndrome

Shy and Drager (1960) described two cases of a neurological syndrome associated with orthostatic hypotension, defective sweating and sphincter disturbances, with the subsequent appearance of somatic neurological manifestations. The pathological changes included widespread degeneration in the medulla, the posterior hypothalamic region, the cerebellum, the third nerve nuclei, the basal ganglia, the autonomic ganglia, the dorsal nucleus of the vagus, with reduction in the number of cells in the anterolateral column of the spinal cord.

Thomas and Schirger (1963) described 30 cases of the syndrome in which the presenting feature was postural hypotension. The ages ranged from 42 to 74 years and the condition was three times as common in men than in women. The onset of the somatoneurological manifestations was usually insidious, and followed the known onset of postural hypotension by six months to 20 years. Eleven patients had features resembling Parkinsonism. The clinical signs indicated involvement of the corticobulbar and corticospinal tracts, the basal ganglia and the cerebellar system. The prognosis was poor.

Bannister (1971) showed that in nearly all patients there was involvement of both cranial and sacral parasympathetic and sympathetic outflows. In the sympathetic nervous system the efferent or central components were more involved than the afferent: and the preganglionic more than the postganglionic.

Parkinsonism

Orthostatic hypotension can occur in patients with paralysis agitans (Barbeau et al, 1969; Aminoff and Wilcox, 1971). The latter authors described 11 patients with Parkinsonism and autonomic dysfunction. Three were cases of the Shy–Drager syndrome in which autonomic symptoms preceded somatic neurological manifestations; while in eight patients the autonomic symptoms succeeded the somatic manifestations. The autonomic manifestations included low resting blood pressure, increased sensitivity to L-noradrenaline, patchy impairment of thermoregulatory sweating, and abnormal bladder function.

Many patients with Parkinsonism prefer a cold to a hot environment but are liable to develop accidental hypothermia (Gubbay and Barwick, 1966). Temperature homeostasis is often impaired (Collins et al, 1977).

Autonomic disturbances in paralysis agitans are often unrecognised. Barbeau and his colleagues (1969) stated that orthostatic hypotension was common in idiopathic Parkinsonism, but Reid et al (1972) and Aminoff and Wilcox (1971) maintained that the circulatory reflexes were usually intact. Gross, Bannister and Godwin-Austen (1972) found that in 20 patients under the age of 63 with idiopathic Parkinsonism the Valsalva responses were normal but the percentage fall in mean blood pressure on passive tilting was significantly greater than in a control group of patients matched for age.

L-Dopa therapy of patients with apparently uncomplicated Parkinsonism sometimes first reveals evidence of autonomic dysfunction.

Cerebrovascular disease

In a geriatric department in Oxford, Johnson and his colleagues (1965) found that a substantial proportion of the patients, many of whom had cerebrovascular disease, suffered from dizziness and an abnormal fall in blood pressure on changing from a lying to a sitting or standing position. In 11 of the 100 patients the systolic pressure fell by 20 mmHg or more after they had sat for 5 min. A similar fall in blood pressure occurred in 17 after they had stood for 2 min. The instability of the blood pressure probably resulted from a lesion in the central nervous system. At autopsy ischaemic lesions were found at many sites in the brain, but not in the spinal cord, hypothalamus or brain-stem. Gross (1970) suggested that age and debility, rather than cerebrovascular disease, might be the important factors.

Orthostatic hypotension and impairment of thermoregulation may also be due to psychotropic drugs, especially phenothiazines, which are commonly used in patients with cerebrovascular disease.

Autonomic neuropathy due to diabetes

Patients with diabetes mellitus may develop symptoms suggestive of autonomic neuropathy; these include, impotence, symptoms of orthostatic hypotension, intermittent nocturnal diarrhoea, intermittent vomiting, gastric fullness or delay in emptying, reduced sweating in the legs and impairment of temperature regulation leading to accidental hypothermia. The incidence of peripheral neuropathy as a complication of diabetes is uncertain. According to Roberts (1970) the reported frequency varies from 4 to 93 per cent. It is even more difficult to estimate the frequency of autonomic involvement. In one series (Rundles, 1945) 25 to 30 per cent of patients with sensory or motor neuropathy were considered to have autonomic neuropathy, and in another series (Odel, Roth and Kealing, 1955) the frequency was greater than 75 per cent.

Sharpey-Schafer and Taylor (1960) first drew attention to the impairment of circulatory reflexes in diabetic neuropathy. Sixty-nine of 337 patients attending a diabetic clinic had evidence of neuropathy. Thirty-five of these were studied fully. Seventeen showed complete absence of circulatory reflexes and 14 a diminution in response to the Valsalva manoeuvre, tipping, coughing, hyperventilation and mental arithmetic. Ewing and his colleagues (1976) found that of 37 patients with clinical features of diabetic autonomic neuropathy one-quarter were dead within 2½ years. Of those who had abnormal autonomic function tests on the first assessment one-half died within the same period. This increased mortality was unrelated to age, duration of diabetes or duration of autonomic symptoms. The authors suggested that in diabetes with clinical features of autonomic neuropathy simple autonomic function tests gave a good guide to prognosis.

Other causes

Other causes of autonomic neuropathy occasionally seen in the elderly include primary amyloidosis and neuropathy associated with malignant disease, especially carcinoma of the bronchus and of the pancreas. Acute polyneuropathy (Guillain–Barré syndrome) sometimes leads to impairment of circulatory reflexes, but the degree of autonomic dysfunction is not related to the extent of motor and sensory involvement.

Wernicke's encephalopathy and other lesions of the hypothalamus

Birchfield (1964) found postural hypotension in 32 of 40 cases of Wernicke's disease. In these 32 patients the other clinical features were ophthalmoparesis (26), nystagmus (32), ataxia (in all of the 25 patients tested), peripheral neuropathy (29) and Korsakoff's psychosis (28). These clinical features were due to metabolic disturbances and to petechial haemorrhages in the hypothalamus resulting from thiamine deficiency, often associated with alcoholism. Since these patients failed to develop reflex vasoconstriction with the Valsalva manoeuvre or cold stimulation, Birchfield considered that the site of the lesion was either the central pathways or the efferent autonomic system. The hypothalamic lesions in Wernicke's encephalopathy can also lead to hypothermia (Philip and Smith, 1973). The disorder of temperature regulation is often overlooked. The response to thiamine administration in Wernicke's encephalopathy is usually dramatic.

Fox and his colleagues (1970, 1973b) have described cases of episodic or intermittent hypothermia associated with other lesions in the hypothalamic region.

Other disorders of the central nervous system

Autonomic dysfunction presenting as orthostatic hypotension or impairment of temperature regulation may occur in a variety of diseases involving the nervous system including tabes dorsalis (Sharpey-Schafer, 1956), Holmes–Adie syndrome (Croll, Duthie and MacWilliam, 1935), paraplegia (Johnson, Park and Frankel, 1971) and chronic alcoholism (Barraclough and Sharpey-Schafer, 1963).

AUTONOMIC REGULATION OF BLOOD PRESSURE

Normal regulation of the circulation

Blood pressure regulation depends on cardiac output and peripheral resistance. Heart rate, which influences cardiac output, is controlled by baroreceptor reflexes originating from the carotid sinus; a fall in blood pressure leads to cardiac acceleration. Peripheral resistance is dependent on vasoconstrictor tone mediated by the sympathetic nervous system. Normally, on standing after lying in the supine position, parasympathetic activity decreases causing cardiac acceleration, and sympathetic activity increases resulting in constriction of arterioles and veins. About 700 ml of blood leaves the chest and is rapidly pooled in the abdomen and legs. The pressure in the right atrium falls to or below the mean intrathoracic pressure and there is diminished return of blood to the right side of the heart. In a fit young adult the systemic arterial pressure drops only transiently on standing, and within 15 to 30 s the pressure has regained the previous level or is a little above it. With more prolonged standing the immediate effects of the neural mechanisms are reinforced by increased secretion of catecholamines from the adrenal medulla and by the liberation of angiotensin and aldosterone.

POSTURAL HYPOTENSION

A fall in blood pressure on standing is common in the elderly and often causes symptoms. In some cases these are so severe as to make an ordinary ambulant life impossible. Lesser degrees of postural hypotension are often unrecognised. In the elderly they are more likely to lead to transient feelings of faintness, giddiness and unsteadiness especially after rising from bed at night or in the morning.

Incidence

Johnson and his co-workers (1965) investigated postural hypotension in patients aged 70 and over admitted to a geriatric department in Oxford. Seventeen per cent of patients had a fall in systolic pressure of 20 mmHg or more on standing for 2 min. Caird and his colleagues (1973) in Glasgow recorded the lying and standing blood pressure of 494 people aged 65 and over living at home. The systolic pressure fell by 20 mmHg or more in 24 per cent of subjects, by 30 mmHg or more in 9 per cent and by 40 mmHg or more in 5 per cent. There was no sex difference, but falls in systolic pressure were significantly more common in those aged 75 and over than in those under that age. The prevalence of postural hypotension in the Glasgow survey was higher than that reported by Rodstein and Zeman (1957) in ambulatory residents in a home for the aged, and by Exton-Smith in old people who participated in a hypothermia survey (Exton-Smith, Green and Fox, 1975; Exton-Smith, 1977).

Pathogenesis

Causes of the increasing incidence of postural hypotension with age include diminished circulatory blood volume in sodium and water deficiency, Addison's disease, or following the continued use of diuretic agents and autonomic dysfunction from age-related decline in physiological mechanisms or from the presence of pathological conditions.

Autonomic dysfunction leading to postural hypotension may be due to impairment of the afferent part of the baroreceptor reflex arc (Sharpey-Schafer and Taylor, 1960), to lesions in the central structures (Appenzeller and Descarries, 1964) or to impairment of function in the effector system (Bannister, Ardill and Fentem, 1967) which is responsible for systemic arteriolar constriction and possibly constriction of venous reservoirs. Wilkins and his colleagues (1951) emphasised that failure to control the splanchnic vascular bed may play an important part in the development of postural hypotension. Low and his co-workers (1975a, b) demonstrated demyelination of the greater splanchnic nerve, which is a major sympathetic pathway, in diabetics with postmortem evidence of peripheral neuropathy and presumed autonomic neuropathy.

Aetiology

The pathological conditions associated with autonomic dysfunction leading to postural hypotension include diabetes, Parkinsonism, cerebrovascular disease, Wernicke's encephalopathy, carcinomatous neuropathy, tabes dorsalis, the Shy–Drager syndrome (see page 87) and the administration of hypotensive drugs, diuretics, L-dopa and the phenothiazines. These conditions are absent in the majority of elderly people with postural hypotension. In the Glasgow study (Caird et al, 1973) two or more of the following factors—varicose veins, urinary tract infections, anaemia, hyponatraemia and potentially hypotensive drugs—were present in 50 per cent of subjects with a fall in systolic pressure of 30 mmHg or more, and in 17 per cent without postural hypotension ($P < 0.01$). This suggests that postural hypotension in relatively healthy old people has more than one cause.

Clinical features

In many instances postural hypotension is asymptomatic; the autoregulation of the cerebral circulation is able to compensate for the fall in systemic arterial pressure. In other cases the patient complains of weakness, faintness, dizziness, loss of balance or blacking out of vision especially when rising from the lying position. Falls associated with postural hypotension may lead to fractures and to accidental hypothermia. When postural hypotension is discovered a search should be made for somatic neurological involvement including peripheral neuropathy, olivo-ponto-cerebellar degeneration, pyramidal tract lesions and Parkinsonism. Overstall and his colleagues (1977) showed that body sway was greater in old people with postural hypotension than in age-matched controls. It seems unlikely that postural hypotension is a common cause of transient cerebral ischaemic attacks (Kendall and Marshall, 1963) or of cerebral infarction.

Management

Appropriate treatment should be given to those patients who are found to have correctable causes of postural hypotension. The use of sympathomimetic drugs has proved disappointing. The administration of fludrocortisone is more promising. This substance expands blood volume, so that even when pooling occurs in the dependent capacity vessels there is sufficient blood to maintain venous return to the heart. The dose given must be large (0.5–2.0 mg/day). In the elderly there is danger of this precipitating congestive cardiac failure or pulmonary oedema. Pooling of blood on assuming the upright position may be prevented by mechanical means, such as the wearing of anti-G trousers, designed primarily for airmen, which is not usually practical in the elderly; or full-length elastic stockings in combination with an elastic abdominal support.

Lang, Jansen and Pfaff (1975) reported significant improvement in postural hypotension treated with dihydroergotamine (2 mg three times a day). Nordenfelt and Mellander (1972) believe that the effects of dihydroergotamine are largely due to its powerful and relatively selective action on the capacity vessels in the peripheral circulation.

DISTURBANCES OF TEMPERATURE REGULATION

NORMAL REGULATION OF BODY TEMPERATURE

For a comprehensive account of the mechanisms of temperature regulation the reader is referred to Fox (1974). Homeothermy, or the capacity to maintain a stable deep body temperature, is an evolutionary development found only in birds, man and other mammals. Ideally in these animals all body tissues would be maintained at optimum temperature, but this would be difficult to achieve and costly in energy production. Thus in man and other homeothermic animals the deep body or 'core' temperature is controlled and the superficial or body 'shell' is used as a variable insulator or heat sink. The heart and circulation act as a heat exchanger system. In a warm environment the blood flow through the skin is increased to promote the transfer of heat to the body surface. Under cool conditions the blood flow is reduced to conserve heat. This vasomotor regulation is capable of maintaining homeothermy only over a narrow range of environmental temperatures. As a protection against hyperthermia and hypothermia the additional mechanisms of sweating and shivering are brought into play. In civilised societies man is able to live almost entirely within the vasomotor control zone without the operation of these emergency mechanisms by adapting his immediate environment through appropriate clothing, heating and air-conditioning.

Thermoregulatory mechanisms

The maintenance of a relatively constant deep body temperature depends upon the balance of heat gain and heat loss from the whole body. The balance is under the control of the nervous system, and in particular of the hypothalamus which is the main thermoregulatory centre of the brain.

Hypothalamic control. The input to the hypothalamic controller comes from the thermosensitive end organs in the skin and from thermosensors mainly within the hypothalamus, particularly in the anterior region. It is probable that the posterior hypothalamus controls the 'set-point' for body temperature regulation. The output from the hypothalamus is mediated through the autonomic effector system controlling peripheral blood flow, shivering, pilo-erection and sweating, and through actions on the endocrine glands and voluntary muscles influencing heat production.

Shivering. Normal metabolic heat production can be increased voluntarily by exercise or involuntarily by a cold environment, producing increased activity in skeletal muscles culminating in shivering. This is mediated through somatic, not autonomic nerves. Shivering is evoked by activity of the cold receptors in the skin, but a fall in central temperature in the hypothalamic region may play a part. At a core body temperature below about 32°C the shivering reaction is abolished and thermogenesis then depends on increase in skeletal muscle tone. Long-term exposure to cold leads to increased output of thyroxine and the catecholamines, adrenaline and noradrenaline.

Vasomotor control. In man vasomotor control in the skin depends upon vasoconstrictor autonomic nerves and on a vasodilator mechanism. The vasoconstrictor mechanism predominates in the hands and the feet and is only weakly represented in the proximal parts of the limbs and the trunk. In a person who feels cold, but who is not shivering, the blood flow in the hands is approximately 1 ml/100 ml of hand tissue/min. Under thermally neutral conditions it is usually in the range of 4 to 10 ml and when the body is heated it rises to over 40 ml (Fox, 1974). The stimulus to vasoconstriction arises mainly from the cold receptors in the skin. Within the vasomotor control zone hand blood flow is very sensitive to small changes in skin temperature in the rest of the body, marked vasoconstriction and vasodilation being elicited by minor degrees of cooling and warming respectively.

The way in which the vasodilator mechanism operates is unknown. Vasodilation occurs over the greater part of the body surface, and may be mediated through the release of the bradykinin-forming enzyme (Fox and Hilton, 1958). Active vasodilation begins just before sweating is initiated, and is the dominant mechanism for promoting heat loss by increasing transport of heat to the skin for evaporation by sweating.

Sweating. Thermoregulatory sweating depends upon the activity of the eccrine glands which are present over most of the skin. They are innervated by postganglionic cholinergic fibres of the sympathetic nervous system. Sweating is initiated by a central receptor mechanism which responds to a rise in deep body temperature, and by reflex activity from thermosensitive receptors in the skin.

ACCIDENTAL HYPOTHERMIA

Hypothermia is defined as a state in which the deep body temperature falls below 35°C (95°F). It became recognised in Great Britain during the 1960s as a problem particularly affecting old people. The term accidental hypothermia is used to imply that the lowering of deep body temperature is unintentional, as distinct from therapeutically induced hypothermia.

INCIDENCE

Until 15 years ago accidental hypothermia in the elderly was thought to be rare. It was known to occur in association with myxoedema, hypopituitarism and alcoholism. The British Medical Association's Committee on Accidental Hypothermia in the Elderly (1964), after reviewing descriptions of cases reported in the literature, concluded that there was no accurate information on the prevalence of the condition. Very few cases were recognised clinically before admission, and elderly people with hypothermia suffered a high mortality.

Hospital studies

Duguid, Simpson and Stowers (1961) described 23 cases occurring in Scotland. All the patients were elderly and developed hypothermia indoors. The deep body temperature on admission, as measured by a rectal thermometer, ranged from 22.8 to 31.9°C. Only seven (30 per cent) of the patients survived. Rosin and Exton-Smith (1964) described 32 patients with hypothermia, half of whom were seen during the very cold winter of 1962/63. With the exception of one aged 39 years their ages ranged from 60 to 92 years. Ten patients were found lying on the floor, 10 were in bed at home, two were sitting in a chair and one developed hypothermia in hospital. The results of a survey in 10 hospital groups during the months February, March and April 1965 showed an incidence of hypothermia in 0.68 per cent of all patients admitted, of whom 42 per cent were aged 65 and over (Royal College of Physicians, 1966). It was estimated that about 3800 elderly patients were admitted with hypothermia to hospitals in Great Britain during these three winter months. Ten years later, a second survey in London, in January to April 1975, showed that 3.6 per cent of patients aged 65 and over who were admitted to hospital were hypothermic, a prevalence considerably higher than that of the previous study.

Population studies

Two small surveys of old people living at home showed that between 5 and 11 per cent had *mouth* temperatures below 35.0°C (Society of Medical Officers of Health, 1968; Williams, 1968). Oral temperature, however, is an unreliable measure of deep body temperature. With the development of the Uritemp technique by Fox and his colleagues (1971) surveys of the elderly population at home became reliable. During the first three months of 1972 the National survey (1020 subjects) and the Camden survey (1000 subjects) revealed that the incidence of deep body temperature below 35.0°C was 0.45 per cent, but an additional 10 per cent of the elderly population were in the 'low' temperature category (35.0–35.5°C Uritemp); that is, they were on the borderline of hypothermia and were considered to be at risk of developing true hypothermia (Fox et al, 1973b). The winter environmental temperature in 1972 was slightly higher than average, but in 75 per cent of cases the room temperature in the morning was 18.3°C or below; and in 10 per cent the room temperature was 12°C or below.

AETIOLOGY

The causes of accidental hypothermia may be grouped under two headings:

Exogenous factors

Exposure to cold is an overriding cause. The Royal College of Physicians' survey (1966) showed a clear relationship between hypothermia and low environmental temperature. The number of cases rose considerably when the ambient temperature fell below 0°C. Exposure is likely to be longer when the old person lives alone and is socially isolated. Many cases, however, occur when the old person is in bed at night apparently well-covered with clothes. In these instances insufficient body heat is being generated, so that even good external insulation is ineffective.

Endogenous factors

Impaired temperature homeostasis. In the national survey (Fox et al, 1973b) the 10 per cent of subjects whose urine temperature was less than 35.5°C were thought to have some degree of thermoregulatory failure, as shown by inability to maintain an adequate core-periphery temperature gradient. The mean difference between the urine temperature and the hand temperature in this group was 2.9°C compared with 4.6°C for those in the 'normal' temperature group whose deep body temperatures were 36.0°C and above. This was confirmed when a subsample were submitted to thermoregulatory function tests using a specially designed air-conditioned bed (Fox, 1975). Shivering occurred during cooling in 12 per cent of the elderly subjects compared with 30 per cent of young adults. Sweating occurred in all the young subjects but in only about half of the elderly during the period of warming. Abnormal peripheral blood flow patterns on cooling and warming were found in 56 per cent of the elderly men and 45 per cent of the women. Of 12 subjects who had deep body temperature below 35.5°C nine had abnormal blood flow patterns, eight failed to sweat on warming and seven had postural hypotension. In only one case was there no evidence of autonomic dysfunction. Autonomic dysfunction was much less frequently seen in 93 subjects who had a normal deep body temperature.

The subjects who participated in the Camden study who were still alive were followed up four years later (Collins et al, 1977). A significantly higher proportion had a resting peripheral blood flow of less than 5 ml/100 ml hand tissue/min and a non-constrictor response on cooling, while in the group with normal peripheral blood flow there was a significant increase in the deep body temperature required to initiate sweating. These studies in the Camden volunteers have established, both on a cross-sectional and longitudinal basis, that there is an age-related decline in autonomic function which leads to impairment of thermoregulatory capacity in a high proportion of old people. These findings suggest that physiological impairment of temperature regulation is one of the factors accounting for an increased risk of hypothermia in the elderly. Macmillan and his colleagues (1967) demonstrated in the survivors of accidental hypothermia that resting deep body temperature was lower and fell abnormally in response to cold in comparison with age-matched controls.

Clinical disorders. Almost any serious illness in an older person can cause hypothermia, but those commonly found include myxoedema, hypopituitarism, diabetes, cerebrovascular accidents, Parkinsonism, mental impairment, confusional states, severe infections, circulatory disturbances and drugs acting on the nervous system, particularly the phenothiazine tranquillisers, sedatives, antidepressive agents and alcohol.

CLINICAL FEATURES

Descriptions of the clinical features are given by Duguid and her colleagues (1961) and by Rosin and Exton-Smith (1964).

Appearance. If there is intense peripheral vasoconstriction the patient is pale. The skin is very cold to touch, even in those parts which are usually covered, for example, the axillae and the abdominal wall. The puffy facial appearance, the slow cerebration and the husky voice may be mistaken for myxoedema.

Level of consciousness. When the body temperature falls below 32°C clouding of consciousness and drowsiness are usually apparent. The lower the body temperature the more likely is the patient to be comatose. In the series described by Rosin and Exton-Smith

(1964) three-quarters of the patients whose rectal temperatures were less than 27°C were unconscious.

Central nervous system. The reflexes are sluggish. The muscular hypertonus which replaces shivering at low temperatures gives rise to neck stiffness simulating meningism and to rigidity of the abdominal wall. An involuntary flapping tremor of the arms and legs has been observed in some patients (Rosin and Exton-Smith, 1964).

Cardiovascular system. The heart rate slows in response to cold, due to sinus bradycardia or slow atrial fibrillation. The electrocardiogram usually shows some degree of heart block, with an increase in PR interval in patients with sinus rhythm and there is delay in intraventricular conduction. A pathognomonic sign is the appearance of a 'J' wave, shown by a characteristic deflection at the junction of the QRS and ST segment (Osborn, 1953; Emslie-Smith, 1958). The size of these waves varies from patient to patient and they are not related to the severity of the hypothermia. They are often absent altogether. The height of the wave diminishes as the deep body temperature rises. A fall in arterial blood pressure is an ominous sign.

Respiratory system. Respiration is slow and shallow. When the hypopnoea is severe a fall in arterial oxygen saturation occurs with consequent anoxia of the tissues (McNicol and Smith, 1964). Bronchopneumonia may be present without the usual clinical signs. Basal crepitations may be due to cold injury to the alveoli.

Alimentary system. Acute pancreatitis is often found at postmortem examination. A rise in the serum amylase was found in 11 of the 15 cases tested by Duguid et al (1961) and in 9 out of 11 cases in our series. Fulminating pancreatitis, a condition generally accompanied by pain and shock, may give rise to few signs in the hypothermic patient. It should be suspected if the patient winces when firm pressure is applied to the epigastrium.

MANAGEMENT

Rapid rewarming of the elderly person suffering from hypothermia is hazardous. If, however, the temperature is allowed to rise slowly and spontaneously the period of hypothermia is greatly prolonged, and irreversible changes in the tissues may take place. In the absence of more satisfactory methods of warming the body core without the application of external heat, one of two therapeutic regimes is advocated.

Mild to moderate hypothermia (32–35°C). The room temperature in a cubicle is maintained at about 27°C to allow the deep body temperature to rise at a rate of about 0.5°/h. The patient is barrier-nursed and a broad-spectrum antibiotic is administered in an attempt to prevent bronchopneumonia. Oxygen is given if tissue anoxia is present. The pulse and blood pressure must be monitored, and if there is a drop in pressure during the course of treatment the patient is cooled again temporarily by lowering the room temperature.

Severe hypothermia (deep body temperature less than 32°C). The patient must be treated in an intensive care unit. The additional measures required are: institution of positive pressure ventilation; insertion of a central venous catheter for the measurement of pressure and for the administration of warm fluids; correction of dehydration and acidosis; and the monitoring of deep body temperature either continuously (by a thermistor in the external auditory meatus) or half-hourly (by a rectal thermometer).

Many patients treated with these regimes regain a normal deep body temperature within 12 to 24 h, but the later outcome is dependent on the degree and duration of the hypothermia and on the nature and severity of the causative clinical condition.

HEAT STROKE AND HEAT-AGGRAVATED ILLNESS

The number of deaths from all causes provides a more valid measure of the effects of extremes of temperature than the numbers revealed by death certification as due to heat illness or hypothermia. The adverse effects of high environmental temperatures are seen mainly in the elderly population, and mortality in the older age groups increases dramatically during heat waves.

Mortality in heat-waves

The United States Vital Statistics Reports for the Nation for the years 1952 to 1967 revealed that during heat-waves persons over the age of 50 showed an increase in deaths from all causes beyond the numbers expected, and progressively so with advancing years (Ellis, 1972). In the heat-waves in New York City in July 1972 and in August and September 1973 excess deaths in the aged population were ascribed mainly to ischaemic heart disease and, to a lesser extent, to cerebrovascular disease (Ellis, Nelson and Pincus, 1975). Only a small proportion of deaths were certified as due to the effects of heat illness alone. In a large home for the aged in Sydney mortality was lowest when the afternoon temperature was between 21 and 26°C, but was 13 per cent above average when the temperature ranged between 27 and 32°C (Macpherson, Ofner and Welch, 1967). This effect of temperature became more marked in persons over the age of 70.

In the more moderate climate of England and Wales mortality also changes with fluctuations in environmental temperature (*OPCS Monitor*, 1975, 1976). It is lowest when the mean temperature is about 17 to 18°C and rises with mean temperatures above about 20°C. These variations are obscured when monthly patterns of mortality are studied because when a heat-wave leads to a sudden increase in mortality of those at greatest risk, fewer die in the immediately succeeding weeks (Lyster, 1976).

The adverse effects of heat-waves are also seen in old people who develop heat stroke. Levine (1969) has described the clinical features of 25 fatal cases among 200 patients who presented in an emergency ward during the heat-wave experienced in New York City in July 1966. The average age was 78.4 years and only three patients were less than 70 years old.

Aetiology

Impairment of thermoregulatory function due to diminished or absent sweating is thought to be one of the factors responsible for the occurrence of heat-stroke and for the increased mortality in the elderly population during heat-waves (Ellis et al, 1976). Foster and his colleagues (1976) investigated the sweating responses to thermal stimulation and to the intradermal injection of acetylcholine or methacholine in 28 men and 18 women aged 70 and over compared with the responses in young subjects. In the old people there was a marked reduction in sweating activity and an increase in the threshold for sweating, which were more pronounced in women. In addition the high incidence of cardiovascular and cerebrovascular disease in elderly people could account for their increased vulnerability to heat; while Ellis (1975) has drawn attention to the dangers during heat-waves of phenothiazines which interfere with thermoregulation and suppress sweating.

Clinical features of heat-stroke in the aged

In the series of 25 fatal cases described by Levine (1969) the average rectal temperature on admission was 41.3°C. Common accompanying conditions included arteriosclerotic heart disease, congestive cardiac failure, diabetes mellitus, Parkinsonism and recent or old stroke. A history of the prodromal phase was rarely available, but some patients complained of weakness, nausea, vomiting, dizziness, headache, breathlessness, anorexia and a feeling of warmth. Important clinical features were dehydration with anhydrosis in the majority of patients (84 per cent), coma with complete unresponsiveness to painful stimuli (72 per cent), and signs of pulmonary consolidation (76 per cent) often due to Gram-negative staphylococcal infection. Six of the 15 patients in whom the serum sodium was estimated had levels above 150 mEq/litre and 8 of 22 patients had serum chloride levels of more than 105 mEq/litre. Elderly patients differ from younger in their ability to combat dehydration because of depressed sensorium, weakness, and failure of the cardiovascular and renal mechanisms for water conservation. The transfer of heat from the body core to the periphery is dependent on circulatory adjustments which are deficient in old people with cardiovascular disease.

Management

The reduction of deep body temperature is usually achieved by cold water sponges and iced baths. Rapid external cooling requires vigorous massage to the skin to counteract rapid reflex peripheral vasoconstriction produced by the markedly elevated core-to-shell thermal gradient induced by external cooling. Circulatory shock occurs in many heat-stroke victims. Steroids are of doubtful value. Intravenous fluids are required to counteract water and/or salt depletion but there is considerable danger of precipitating pulmonary oedema. The prognosis is very poor due to serious underlying disease.

REFERENCES

Aminoff, M. J. & Wilcox, C. S. (1971) Assessment of autonomic function in patients with a Parkinsonian syndrome. *British Medical Journal*, **iv**, 80–84.

Appenzeller, O. & Descarries, L. (1964) Circulatory reflexes in patients with cerebrovascular disease. *New England Journal of Medicine*, **271**, 820–823.

Bannister, R. G. (1971) Degeneration of the autonomic nervous system. *Lancet*, **ii**, 175–179.

Bannister, R., Ardill, L. & Fentem, P. (1967) Defective autonomic control of blood vessels in idiopathic orthostatic hypotension. *Brain*, **90**, 725–746.

Barbeau, A., Gillo-Joffroy, L., Bouchier, R., Nowaczynski, W. & Genest, J. (1969) Reninaldosterone system in Parkinson's disease. *Science*, **165**, 291–292.

Barraclough, M. A. & Sharpey-Schafer, E. P. (1963) Hypotension from absent circulatory reflexes: effects of alcohol, barbiturates, psychotherapeutic drugs and other mechanisms. *Lancet*, **i**, 1121–1126.

Birchfield, R. I. (1964) Postural hypotension in Wernicke's disease. *American Journal of Medicine*, **36**, 404–414.

Bowen, D. M., White, P., Flack, R. H. A., Smith, C. B. & Davison, A. N. (1974) Brain decarboxylase activities as indices of pathological change in senile dementia. *Lancet*, **i**. 1247.

Bristow, J. C., Gribbon, B., Honour, A. J., Pickering, T. G. & Sleight, P. (1969) Diminished baroreflex sensitivity in high blood pressure and aging man. *Journal of Physiology*, **202**, 45–46P.

British Medical Association Memorandum (1964) Accidental hypothermia in the elderly. *British Medical Journal*, **ii**, 1255–1258.

Caird, F. I., Andrews, G. R. & Kennedy, R. D. (1973) Effect of posture on blood pressure in the elderly. *British Heart Journal*, **35**, 527–530.

Collins, K. J., Dore, C., Exton-Smith, A. N., Fox, R. H., MacDonald, I. C. & Woodward, P. M. (1977). Accidental hypothermia and impaired temperature homeostasis in the elderly. *British Medical Journal* **i**, 353–356.

Croll, W. F., Duthie, R. J. & MacWilliam, J. A. (1935) Postural hypotension: report of a case. *Lancet*, **i**, 194–198.

Duguid, H., Simpson, R. G. & Stowers, J. M. (1961) Accidental hypothermia. *Lancet*, **ii**, 1213–1219.

Ellis, F. P. (1972) Mortality from heat illness and heat-aggravated illness in the United States. *Environmental Research*, **5**, 1–58.

Ellis, F. P. (1976) Heat waves and drugs affecting temperature regulation. *British Medical Journal*, **iii**, 474.

Ellis, F. P., Exton-Smith, A. N., Foster, K. G. & Weiner, J. S. (1976) Mortality during heat waves in very young and very old persons and eccrine sweating. *Israel Journal of Medical Science*, **12**, 111–116.

Ellis, F. P., Nelson, F. & Pincus, L. (1975) Mortality during heat waves in New York City, July 1972 and August–September, 1973. *Environmental Research*, **10**, 1–13.

Emslie-Smith, D. (1958) Accidental hypothermia: a common condition with a pathognomonic ECG. *Lancet*, **ii**, 492–495.

Ewing, D. J., Campbell, I. W. & Clarke, B. F. (1976) Mortality in diabetic autonomic neuropathy. *Lancet*, **i**, 601–603.

Exton-Smith, A. N. (1977) Functional consequences of ageing: clinical manifestations. In *Care of the Elderly: Meeting the Challenge of Dependency*, ed. Exton-Smith, A. N. & Grimley Evans, J. London: Academic Press.

Exton-Smith, A. N., Green, M. F. & Fox, R. H. (1975) An intensive study of elderly people with particular reference to control of body temperature. In *Proceedings of the 10th International Congress of Gerontology*, Jerusalem.

Foster, K. G., Ellis, F. P., Dore, C., Exton-Smith, A. N. & Weiner, J. S. (1976) Sweat responses in the aged. *Age and Ageing*, **5**, 91–101.

Fox, R. H. (1974) Temperature regulation with special reference to man. In *Recent Advances in Physiology*, ed. Linden, R. J. London: Churchill Livingstone.

Fox, R. H. (1975) Hypothermia, heating and the elderly: physiological aspects. *Centre for Environmental Studies Symposium*, London.

Fox, R. H., Davies, T. W., Marsh, F. P. & Urich, H. (1970) Hypothermia in a young man with an anterior hypothalamic lesion. *Lancet*, **ii**, 185–188.

Fox, R. H. & Hilton, S. M. (1958) Bradykinin formation in human skin as a factor in heat vasodilatation. *Journal of Physiology*, **142**, 219–232.

Fox, R. H., Wilkins, D. C., Bell, J. A. et al (1973a) Spontaneous periodic hypothermia: diencephalic epilepsy. *British Medical Journal*, **ii**, 693–695.

Fox, R. H., Woodward, P. M., Exton-Smith, A. N., Green, M. F., Donnison, D. V. & Wicks, M. H. (1973b) Body temperatures in the elderly: a national study of physiological, social and environmental conditions. *British Medical Journal*, **i**, 200–206.

Fox, R. H., Woodward, P. M., Fry, A. J., Collins, J. C. & MacDonald, I. C. (1971) Diagnosis of accidental hypothermia of the elderly. *Lancet*, **i**, 424–427.

Frolkis, V. V., Bezrukov, V. V., Duplenko, Y. P., Shchegoleva, I. V., Shevtchnk, V. G. & Verkhratsky, N. S. (1973) Acetylcholine metabolism and cholinergic regulation of functions in aging. *Gerontologia*, **19**, 45–54.

Gross, M. (1970) Circulatory reflexes in cerebral ischaemia involving different vascular territories. *Clinical Science*, **38**, 491–502.

Gross, M., Bannister, R. & Godwin-Austen, R. (1972) Orthostatic hypotension in Parkinson's disease. *Lancet*, **i**, 174–176.

Gubbay, S. S. & Barwick, D. D. (1966) Two cases of accidental hypothermia in Parkinson's disease with unusual EEG findings. *Journal of Neurology, Neurosurgery and Psychiatry*, **29**, 459–466.

Johnson, R. H., Smith, A. C., Spalding, J. M. K. & Wollner, L. (1965) Effect of posture on blood pressure in elderly patients. *Lancet*, **i**, 731–733.

Johnson, R. H., Park, D. M. & Frankel, H. L. (1971) Orthostatic hypotension and the reninangiotensin system in paraplegia. *Paraplegia*, **9**, 146–152.

Kendall, R. E. & Marshall, J. (1963) Role of hypotension in the genesis of transient focal cerebral ischaemic attacks. *British Medical Journal*, **ii**, 344–348.

Lang, E., Jansen, W. & Pfaff, W. (1975) Orthostatische hypotenie bei älteren menschen. *Medizinische Klinik*, **70**, 1979–1981.

Levine, J. A. (1969) Heat stroke in the aged. *American Journal of Medicine*, **47**, 251–257.

Low, P. A., Walsh, J. C., Huang, C. Y. & McLeod, J. G. (1975a) Sympathetic nervous system in diabetic neuropathy—a clinical and pathological study. *Brain*, **98**, 341–356.

Low, P. A., Walsh, J. C., Huang, C. Y. & McLeod, J. G. (1975b) Sympathetic nervous system in alcoholic neuropathy—a clinical and pathological study. *Brain*, **98**, 357–364.

Lyster, W. R. (1976) Death in summer. *Lancet*, **ii**, 469.

Macmillan, A. L., Corbett, J. L., Johnson, R. H., Smith, A. C., Spalding, J. M. K. & Wollner, L. (1967) Temperature regulation in survivors of accidental hypothermia of the elderly. *Lancet*, **ii**, 165–169.

McNicol, M. W. & Smith, R. (1964) Accidental hypothermia. *British Medical Journal*, **i**, 19–21.

Macpherson, R. K., Ofner, F. & Welch, J. A. (1967) Effect of prevailing air temperature on mortality. *British Journal of Preventive and Social Medicine*, **21**, 1–17.

Nordenfelt, I. & Mellander, S. (1972) Central haemodynamic effects of dihydroergotamine in patients with orthostatic hypotension. *Acta medica scandinavica*, **191**, 115.

Odel, H. M., Roth, G. M. & Kealing, F. R. (1955) Autonomic neuropathy simulating the effects of sympathectomy as a complication of diabetes mellitus. *Diabetes*, **4**, 92–98.

OPCS Monitor (1975, 1976) London: Office of Population Censuses and Surveys.

Osborn, J. J. (1953) Experimental hypothermia: respiratory and blood pH changes in relation to cardiac function. *American Journal of Physiology*, **175**, 389–398.

Overstall, P. W., Imms, F. J., Exton-Smith, A. N. & Johnson, A. L. (1977) Falls in the elderly related to postural imbalance. *British Medical Journal* **i**, 261–264.

Philip, G. & Smith, J. F. (1973) Hypothermia and Wernicke's encephalopathy. *Lancet*, **ii**, 122–124.

Reid, J. L., Calne, D. B., George, C. F. & Vakil, S. D. (1972) The action of L-dopa on baroreflexes in Parkinsonism. *Clinical Science*, **43**, 851–859.

Roberts, A. H. (1970) Neurological complications of systemic diseases. *British Medical Journal*, **i**, 33–35.

Rodstein, M. & Zeman, F. D. (1957) Postural blood pressure changes in the elderly. *Journal of Chronic Diseases*, **6**, 581–588.

Rosin, A. & Exton-Smith, A. N. (1964) Clinical features of accidental hypothermia with observations on thyroid function. *British Medical Journal*, **i**, 16–19.

Royal College of Physicians of London (1966) *Report of Committee on Accidental Hypothermia*.

Rundles, R. W. (1945) Diabetic neuropathy: general review with report of 125 cases. *Medicine*, **24**, 111–160.

Sharpey-Schafer, E. P. (1956) Circulatory reflexes in chronic disease of the afferent nervous system. *Journal of Physiology*, **134**, 1–10.

Sharpey-Schafer, E. P. & Taylor, P. J. (1960) Absent circulatory reflexes in diabetic neuritis. *Lancet*, **i**, 559–562.

Shy, G. M. & Drager, G. A. (1960) A neurological syndrome associated with orthostatic hypotension. *Archives of Neurology*, **2**, 511–527.

Society of Medical Officers of Health, Hypothermia Subcommittee of the Welfare Group (1968) *Public Health (London)*, **82**, 223–227.

Strandell, T. (1964) Circulatory studies in healthy old men. *Acta medica scandinavica*, **175**, Suppl. **414**, 1–44.

Thomas, J. E. & Schirger, A. (1963) Neurologic manifestations in idiopathic orthostatic hypotension. *Archives of Neurology*, **8**, 204–208.

Thomas, J. E. & Schirger, A. (1970) Idiopathic orthostatic hypotension. *Archives of Neurology*, **22**, 289–293.

Thorner, M. O. (1975) Dopamine is an important neurotransmitter in the autonomic nervous system. *Lancet*, **i**, 662–664.

Wilkins, R. W., Culbertson, J. W. & Ingelfinger, F. L. (1951) Effect of splanchnic sympathectomy in hypertensive patients. *Journal of Clinical Investigation*, **30**, 312–319.

Williams, B. T. (1968) Oral temperatures of elderly applicants for welfare services. *Gerontologia clinica*, **10**, 281–287.

7. The interpretation of biochemical data

H. M. Hodkinson

Biochemical investigation of the elderly gives rise to many special problems. First there are problems due to uncertainty about normal ranges in old age. Next, there are problems in the investigation of patients whose test results are upset by the non-specific effects of severe illness, by the influence of multiple disease processes and by the effects of drugs given as treatment. Finally, clinical diagnosis is often very difficult in old age because of the frequency of the atypical presentation of disease (Hodkinson, 1973a). Biochemical investigation based on a screening approach rather than on the usual 'discretionary' application of tests (Holland and Whitehead, 1974) is therefore necessary if treatable conditions such as osteomalacia, myxoedema or thyrotoxicosis are not to be missed when the clinical picture is unusual. Unfortunately, the screening method of using tests gives rise to many more difficulties in interpretation than does discretionary use.

NORMAL RANGES IN OLD AGE

The determination of normal ranges for biochemical tests appropriate to the elderly has been delayed for several reasons. The elderly are a relatively neglected group, and have not been extensively investigated, nor have they been considered of great academic interest. There are difficulties in finding normal ranges in the age group. It is not difficult to find younger subjects who can be regarded as clinically normal, but in old age a totally normal individual is an intellectual abstraction.

Groups of blood donors have been a fruitful source of study for determination of ranges and for the elucidation of age and sex effects (Roberts, 1967; Keating et al, 1969; Flynn et al, 1974) but do not include subjects aged 65 and over. Such studies have shown that in a considerable number of biochemical determinations statistically significant age or sex differences occur, although in most cases the differences are too small to be of clinical importance. Information about subjects aged 65 and over has depended on the study of community samples.

Normal ranges in the elderly have been reviewed by Caird (1973) and by Hyams (1973). In the important study of Leask, Andrews and Caird (1973) 16 biochemical tests were applied to almost 500 elderly subjects in the community. The range for electrolytes, magnesium and bilirubin was the same as in younger adults. In the ranges for total protein, albumin, globulin, calcium and phosphate there were minor but statistically significant age changes (Roberts, 1967; Keating et al, 1969). Phosphate levels in elderly males were considerably lower than in females (Hodkinson, 1973b).

Thyroid function tests

The in vitro thyroid function tests (protein-bound iodine, T4, T3 uptake, free-thyroxine index and TSH) have been studied in elderly community samples by Thomson and his colleagues (1972), Taylor, Thomson and Caird (1974) and Hodkinson, and Denham (1977). The normal range for free-thyroxine index in the elderly is much the same as that for younger ages, but modest elevation of TSH (up to 20 μU/litre) is fairly common in euthyroid elderly subjects.

Random blood glucose levels tend to rise with age (Thomas and Whitehead, 1974). There has been much discussion as to whether this represents an age change or indicates an increasing prevalence of diabetes. The work of Denham (1972b) and Caird (1973) supports the latter view.

Other biochemical tests show high ranges in old age; examples are urea, creatinine, uric acid, cholesterol and alkaline phosphatase (Leask et al, 1973).

Urea and creatinine

The blood levels of urea reflect a balance between endogenous production and renal excretion. Whilst urea production tends to fall with age, glomerular filtration rate (GFR) falls more strikingly (Davies and Shock, 1950). Similar considerations apply to creatinine, although the very low endogenous production associated with the low muscle mass of very small old women may give unexpectedly low creatinine values (Bahemuka et al, 1974). Denham, Hodkinson and Fisher (1975) showed that serum urea and creatinine values were independent of age when variations in GFR and body size were taken into account.

Cholesterol levels are raised in old age (Leask et al, 1973), although they may be lowered in advanced old age by poor nutrition or illness (Denham, 1972a).

Alkaline phosphatase has been widely reported as having a higher range in old age (Chen and Millard, 1972; Sharland, 1972; Leask et al, 1973). There is uncertainty as to whether this is a true change or whether it represents the inclusion of subjects with occult disease. Hodkinson and McPherson (1973) showed that there were many causes of raised alkaline phosphatase in elderly patients. When these were carefully excluded, the range for alkaline phosphatase in the elderly was no higher than that in younger subjects.

Occult disease

Whether higher ranges in the elderly are true age changes or are due to occult disease is not merely academic. If elevated values are wrongly attributed to age, the usefulness of the test in the recognition of potentially treatable disease is diminished. Conversely, failure to appreciate that elevation is an age effect may result in unnecessary investigation of elderly patients.

DISTURBANCE OF NORMAL RANGES

Knowledge of normal ranges based on the study of well old people is necessary for the rational interpretation of biochemical results, but is inadequate when dealing with severely ill dehydrated elderly patients with impaired renal function and multiple diseases and in receipt of a number of drugs.

Dehydration

In the presence of dehydration which is common in elderly patients, urea and creatinine levels are elevated and become unreliable guides to renal function (Bahemuka et al, 1974). Dehydration also gives rise to elevated values or conceals previously low values of other blood components such as sodium and plasma proteins.

Cuffing effects

Venepuncture in ill dehydrated old people is difficult because of collapsed, thin-walled and excessively mobile veins. Prolonged cuffing may be necessary to obtain a blood specimen, but this leads to concentration of macromolecules to which the vein wall is impermeable. Measurements of protein and of protein-bound substances such as calcium are misleadingly high. Cuffing effects are of practical importance in geriatric inpatient practice (Hodkinson, 1973c).

Severe illness

Severe illness may lower levels of protein, particularly of albumin and total iron-binding capacity (Hodkinson, 1975) and of thyroxine-binding globulin, reflected by decreased T3-uptake values (Jefferys et al, 1972). These changes are probably due to impaired protein synthesis occurring as a consequence of constitutional disturbance (Hodkinson, 1975). As these are carrier proteins, severe illness may distort the results for protein-bound substances. It is necessary to correct calcium values in elderly patients for albumin variation, a factor of 0.018 mmol/litre calcium per g/litre of albumin being appropriate (Hodkinson, 1975). Calculation of the free-thyroxine index overcomes the problem of alterations of thyroxine-binding globulin (Jefferys et al, 1972).

Renal impairment

Renal impairment is common in elderly hospital patients, as is shown by the 95 per cent range of 3 to 21 mmol/litre for urea in inpatients (Hodkinson, 1973c). Renal impairment produces enough raised phosphate results sufficient to skew to the right the distribution for inpatients (Hodkinson, 1973b). The test is an unreliable guide to the diagnosis of osteomalacia unless renal function is adequate. Bicarbonate and potassium results may also be seriously disturbed by renal impairment (Hodkinson, 1973c). Uric acid levels may rise when renal function is poor. The test needs to be interpreted with caution.

Alkaline phosphatase

The value of the alkaline phosphatase test in the diagnosis of osteomalacia is seriously reduced, because liver disease, bone trauma, Paget's disease and rheumatoid arthritis all occur more commonly as causes of high levels in geriatric practice (Hodkinson and McPherson, 1973).

Enzymes

The value of enzyme elevation in the confirmation of a diagnosis of myocardial infarction in elderly patients is dubious. Elevation of HBD or LDH may be due to megaloblastic anaemia; elevation of HBD, SGOT or CPK may be associated with stroke (Denham and Hodkinson, 1973); while elevation of SGOT and HBD may be due to liver disorders.

Drugs

Drugs are an important cause of abnormal biochemical results in the elderly. The abnormalities may be due to known pharmacological effects, for example hyponatraemia from diuretics, hypoglycaemia from oral antidiabetic drugs or hypercalcaemia due to vitamin D. Abnormalities may also be due to side-effects, for example hyperuricaemia associated with thiazide diuretics, enzyme elevation due to hepatotoxicity from phenothiazine tranquillisers, or abnormal thyroid function tests due to alterations of thyroxine-binding globulin levels by sex hormones or anabolic hormone. Some less well-known side-effects in elderly patients are severe hyponatraemia as complicating chlorpropamide treatment or hypocalcaemia and hypophosphataemia as a side-effect of oestrogen therapy or of intravenous glucose infusions. Osteomalacia may be suspected. Elevated values of free-thyroxine index often occur after each dose of L-dopa (Hodkinson, 1974). Digitalis and cotrimoxazole may also have this effect (Baruch, Davis and Hodkinson, 1976).

Drugs may produce abnormalities because of analytical interference. The elevation of protein-bound iodine which is due to iodine-containing drugs or contrast media is familiar. Other effects are reviewed by Walker (1974).

Nutrition

Dietary intake affects the levels of ascorbic acid, folate, vitamin D and cholesterol (Denham, 1972a). The time interval since the last meal affects many biochemical measurements. This source of variation is removed by standardising the time of venepuncture and its relationship to the last meal while diurnal variation is also minimised.

SCREENING

'Screening' means the use of tests without a specific clinical indication (Holland and Whitehead, 1974). The frequent atypical presentation in elderly patients of important treatable conditions such as osteomalacia and thyroid disease makes screening attractive.

Screening for occult disease implies the use of multiple tests. Increasing automation in biochemical laboratory work has encouraged the widespread use of multiphasic biochemical profiles. The profile is more economical than a smaller number of discretionary tests. The clinician investigating elderly patients is thus likely to use a hospital admission profile of tests whose purpose is in part for screening and in part discretionary. A profile is difficult to interpret even when normal ranges have been determined, and when disturbing factors are recognised.

The concept of 'normal range'

The term 'normal range' refers to the normal (Gaussian) distribution and not to normal in the sense of non-pathological. The normal distribution together with the closely related log-normal distribution (where a normal distribution is obtained when the observed values are replaced by their logarithms) adequately describe virtually all populations of biochemical measurements encountered in clinical practice (Flynn et al, 1974). The normal distribution can be described by two parameters, the mean and the standard deviation. The distribution has as one of its properties the probability that 95 per cent of the population of measurements will lie within 1.96 standard deviations of the mean. These two values (mean $\pm$ 1.96 standard deviations) provide the limits of the normal range. When we speak of 'normal range' in clinical practice, we are usually referring to the normal range for the test as derived from a sample of healthy individuals of the appropriate sex and age group.

Single tests

A single test result in a healthy individual has a 95 per cent probability of lying within the normal range and a 5 per cent probability of being classified as 'abnormal'. In screening for a disease with a low prevalence of say 2 per cent, an 'abnormal' result is more likely to come from a healthy person than from one with the disease.

Multiple tests

With multiple tests the probability of obtaining a 'normal' set of results falls as the number of tests increases—77 per cent for five tests, 60 per cent for 10 and 35 per cent for 20. Table 7.1 gives further details of sampling expectations for multiple tests.

Table 7.1 Sampling expectations for independent tests

Number of tests performed	Expected percentage of cases with stated number of tests results outside normal limits				
	0	1	2	3	4
5	77.4	20.4	2.1	0.1	0.0
10	59.9	31.5	7.5	1.0	0.1
15	46.3	36.6	13.5	3.1	0.5
20	35.2	37.7	18.9	6.0	1.3
25	27.7	36.5	23.1	9.3	2.7
30	21.5	34.0	25.9	12.7	4.5
50	7.7	20.2	26.1	22.0	13.6

It is difficult for clinicians to cope with the volume of results generated by biochemical profiles (Whitehead and Wootton, 1974). They often fail to act on many abnormal results (Bates and Yellin, 1972).

Pattern recognition with the use of normal ranges has been advocated as a way of meeting these difficulties—'looking at a body of results as a gestalt—an integrated whole rather than a series of disparate, uncoordinated single results' (Reece, 1974). This has had very limited success. The combinatorial aspect seems to have proved theoretical rather than practical. The 'normal range' approach is inadequate to deal with multiphasic profile results.

An alternative approach for screening tests

When a screening test is applied to a group of people a proportion of whom have a disease, the results form two normal (or log-normal) populations. There is overlap between the results from the larger healthy population and those from the smaller diseased one, as shown in Figure 7.1. An example of random glucose values and diabetes was shown by Denham (1972b). In the figure, two values of the test are marked 'a'—at which the probability (given by the height under the curve) of having and of not having the disease is equal —and 'b'—the upper limit of normal for the population without the disease. The former value, termed the critical limit (Murphy and Abbey, 1967), is the best value for the classification of test results as 'normal' and 'abnormal'. A test value above the critical limit indicates a greater than 50 per cent probability of the disease. The critical limit affords a more rational basis for classification in screening than does the normal limit.

The critical limit

The determination of the critical limit requires the following:

1. Distribution of test values for the disease-free population and knowledge of its size.
2. Distribution of test values for the population having the disease and its size.

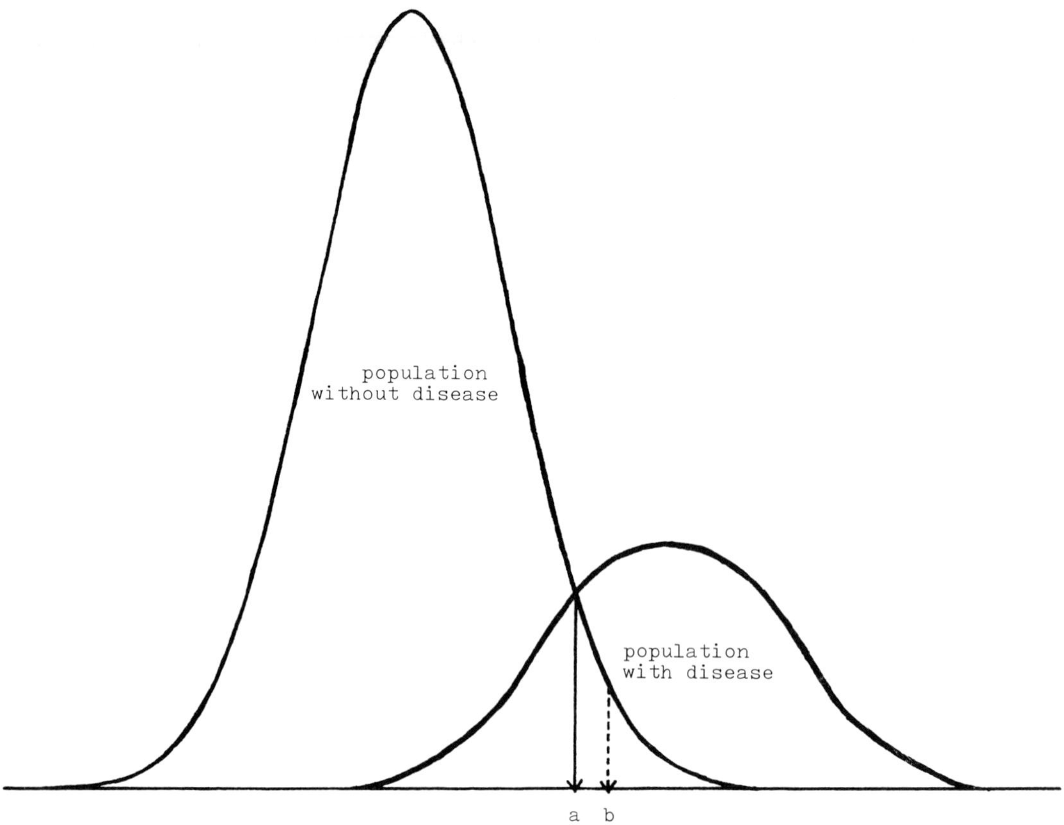

Fig. 7.1 Distributions of test values for populations with and without a disease showing the critical limit (a) and normal limit (b)

The critical limit refers to the local situation. Different critical limits obtain where populations differ.

The critical limit as so far considered implies that positive and negative classification errors have equal weight. The critical limit can be weighted to give an increased cost to false negative classifications, by scaling up the size of the disease population by the required factor and redetermining the crossover point (Murphy and Abbey, 1967).

The critical limit and multiple tests

The critical limit can be applied where more than one test is used at the same time, provided that the rests can be combined to give a single numerical value. Thus, T4-and T3-

uptake results can be combined as the free-thyroxine index to which the critical limit approach can be applied (Hodkinson, 1977).

The discriminant function

The discriminant function is the sum of test values, each multiplied by a signed weighting factor derived from the analysis of previous cases in such a way as to achieve maximum separation of the distribution of the function in disease and non-disease groups. Weiner and Marmorston (1969) showed that linear discriminant functions can be used to derive a single value to which critical limits can be applied.

Discriminant function analysis is complex. Computer programs are available. Clinicians are reluctant to use this despite its great potential value. It has been applied to the diagnosis of thyroid disease (Barnett et al, 1973) and to osteomalacia in a geriatric unit (Hodkinson, 1977).

Discriminant function analysis can also be applied to groups of tests used to separate several disease categories. The value of this application has been demonstrated in the differential diagnosis of hypercalcaemia in adults (Fraser et al, 1971) and in elderly hospital patients (Grero and Hodkinson, 1976).

CONCLUSION

As more biochemical tests become available, previously concealed difficulties in investigation become apparent. Barnett and his colleagues comment, 'although the laboratory problems in testing are still formidable, they are being solved far more rapidly than are the problems relating to the medical usefulness of tests' (Barnett, Civin and Schoen, 1970). Investigation of the elderly highlights the problems, and may prove to be a field where clinicians are well placed to meet the challenges posed by new biochemical tests.

REFERENCES

Bahemuka, M., Hodkinson, H. M., Denham, M. J. & Padmore, G. R. A. (1974) Serum creatinine in a geriatric in-patient population. *Age and Ageing*, **3**, 43–48.

Barnett, D. B., Greenfield, A. A., Howlett, P. J., Hudson, J. C. & Smith, R. N. (1973) Discriminant value of thyroid function tests. *British Medical Journal*, **ii**, 144–147.

Barnett, R. N., Civin, W. H. & Schoen, I. (1970) Multiphasic screening by laboratory tests—an overview of the problem. *American Journal of Clinical Pathology*, **54**, 483–489.

Baruch, A. L. H., Davis, C. & Hodkinson, H. M. (1976) Causes of high free-thyroxine index values in sick euthyroid elderly patients. *Age and Ageing*, **5**, 224–227.

Bates, B. & Yellin, J. A. (1972) The yield of multiphasic screening. *Journal of the American Medical Association*, **222**, 74–78.

Caird, F. I. (1973) Problems of interpretation of laboratory findings in the old. *British Medical Journal*, **iv**, 348–351.

Chen, F. W. K. & Millard, P. H. (1972) The effect of ageing on certain biochemical values. *Modern Geriatrics*, **2**, 92–106.

Davies, D. F. & Shock, N. W. (1950) Age changes in the glomerular filtration rate, effective renal plasma flow and tubular excretory capacity. *Journal of Clinical Investigation*, **29**, 496–507.

Denham, M. J. (1972a) Cholesterol as a parameter of subnutrition in the elderly in-patient. *Gerontologia clinica*, **14**, 235–241.

Denham, M. J. (1972b) The value of random blood glucose determinations as a screening method for detecting diabetes mellitus in the elderly in-patient. *Age and Ageing*, **1**, 55–60.

Denham, M. J. & Hodkinson, H. M. (1973) Serum enzymes and prognosis in cerebral infarction. *Age and Ageing*, **2**, 86–91.

Denham, M. J., Hodkinson, H. M. & Fisher, M. (1975) Glomerular filtration rate in sick elderly in-patients. *Age and Ageing*, **4**, 32–36.

Flynn, F. V., Piper, K. A. J., Garcia-Webb, P., Matherson, K. & Healy, M. J. R. (1974). The frequency distributions of commonly determined blood constituents in healthy blood donors. *Clinica chimica acta*, **52**, 163–171.

Fraser, P., Healy, M., Rose, N. & Watson, L. (1971). Discriminant functions in differential diagnosis of hypercalcaemia. *Lancet*, **i**, 1314–1319.

Grero, P. S. & Hodkinson, H. M. (1976) Hypercalcaemia in elderly hospital in-patients: value of discriminant analysis in differential diagnosis. *Age and Ageing*, **6**, 14–20.

Hodkinson, H. M. (1973a) Non-specific presentation of illness. *British Medical Journal*, **iv**, 94–96.

Hodkinson, H. M. (1973b) Serum inorganic phosphate in a geriatric inpatient population. *Gerontologia clinica*, **15**, 45–49.

Hodkinson, H. M. (1973c) Interpretation of biochemical data in the elderly. *British Journal of Hospital Medicine*, **10**, 684–686.

Hodkinson, H. M. (1974) Biochemical side-effects of drugs in the elderly. *Gerontologia clinica*, **16**, 175–178.

Hodkinson, H. M. (1975) *Diagnostic and prognostic aspects of routine laboratory screening of the geriatric in-patient*. D. M. thesis, University of Oxford.

Hodkinson, H. M. (1977) *Biochemical diagnosis of the elderly*. London: Chapman and Hall.

Hodkinson, H. M. & Denham, M. J. (1977) Thyroid function tests in the elderly in the community. *Age and Ageing*, **6**, 67–70.

Hodkinson, H. M. & McPherson, C. K. (1973) Alkaline phosphatase in a geriatric in-patient population. *Age and Ageing*, **2**, 28–33.

Holland, W. W. & Whitehead, T. P. (1974) Value of new laboratory tests in diagnosis and treatment. *Lancet*, **ii**, 291–394.

Hyams, D. E. (1973) The blood. In *Textbook of Geriatric Medicine and Geronotology*, ed. Brocklehurst, J. C., Edinburgh and London: Churchill Livingstone. pp. 528–292.

Jefferys, P. M., Farran, H. E. A., Hoffenberg, R., Fraser, P. M. & Hodkinson, H. M. (1972) Thyroid function tests in the elderly. *Lancet*, **i**, 924–927.

Keating, F. R., Jones, J. D., Elveback, L. R. & Randall, R. V. (1969) The relation of age and sex to distribution of values in healthy adults of serum calcium, inorganic phosphorus, magnesium, alkaline phosphatase, total proteins, albumin and blood urea. *Journal of Laboratory and Clinical Medicine*, **73**, 825–834.

Leask, R. G. S., Andrews, G. R. & Caird, F. I. (1973) Normal values of sixteen blood constituents in the elderly. *Age and Ageing*, **2**, 14–23.

Murphy, E. A. & Abbey, H. (1967) The normal range—a common misuse. *Journal of Chronic Diseases*, **20**, 79–85.

Reece, R. L. (1974) Using a computer to interpret multiphasic screening results. *Geriatrics*, **29**, 51–91.

Roberts, L. B. (1967) The normal ranges with statistical analysis for seventeen blood constituents. *Clinica chimica acta*, **16**, 69–78.

Sharland, D. E. (1972) Serum alkaline phosphatase; the levels and patterns of isoenzymes in the non-hospitalised elderly. *Age and Ageing*, **1**, 168–176.

Taylor, B. B., Thomson, J. A. & Caird, F. I. (1974) Further studies of thyroid function tests in the elderly at home. *Age and Ageing*, **2**, 122–126.

Thomas, D. J. & Whitehead, T P. (1974) Fasting blood-glucose levels, *Lancet*, **ii**, 900–902.

Thomson, J. A., Andrews, G. R., Caird, F. I. & Wilson, R. (1972) Serum protein bound and plasma inorganic iodine in the elderly at home. *Age and Ageing*, **1**, 158–161.

Walker, G. (1974) Drug interference with chemical tests. *Modern Medicine*, **19**, 197–199.

Weiner, J. M. & Marmorston, J. (1969) Statistical techniques of difference. *Annals of the New York Academy of Sciences*, 161, 641–645.

Whitehead, T. P. & Wootton, I. D. P. (1974) Biochemical profiles in hospital patients. *Lancet*, **ii**, 1439–1443.

8. Principles of drug action and usage

James Williamson

Increasing concern exists in Britain and other developed countries over the escalating costs of drugs and the increasing incidence of their side-effects in the population. It seems that the public commonly expects drugs not only for every disease but even for every symptom and many doctors tend to connive at this. Trethowan (1975) has pointed out that the number of 'central nervous system' drug prescriptions (69.6 millions) in 1972 in England exceeded all other categories and within this group the number of psychoactive drugs (45.3 millions) greatly exceeded any other group. He interpreted this as showing that people not only expect a drug for each symptom but even for each personal problem.

The seriousness increases in older groups for a variety of reasons. First, the numbers of aged persons are increasing. Second, old people tend to have multiple illnesses, symptoms and complaints and their families often may demand that 'something be done'. Third, old people often are subject to social and psychological stress as a result of changes in their status and in society and thus present to their doctors with ill-defined and recurring symptoms arising from loneliness and feelings of alienation or rejection. It is difficult, sometimes impossible, to alleviate these complaints and the hard-pressed doctor may prescribe drugs as a first and last resort. Although this initially may appear to help and may quell the family clamour, it is undoubtedly 'bad medicine'.

Extent of drug use by elderly patients

Exact figures on the amount and nature of the drugs used by the elderly are not available, but recent publications give some idea. One hundred and fifty patients, who comprised all persons aged 75 and over in one practice, were reported by Law and Chalmers (1976). Of these 87 per cent were on *regular* drug therapy, a figure which is three times that for the general population. Thirty-four per cent were taking three or four drugs daily, the common est being analgesics, psychotropics, 'genito-urinary drugs' and cardiac drugs (digitalis and diuretics). Shaw and Opit (1976) investigated the patients aged 70 and over in a Birmingham practice and found that half were on long-term drug therapy, mainly for heart disease, depression and anxiety. Fourteen per cent had had no recorded contact with their GP for six months or longer despite being on continuing medication. Gibson and O'Hare (1968) from the Glasgow Geriatric Service studied 273 patients seen in home visitation: 236 were on drugs, one receiving 13 medications. Twenty-eight per cent received barbiturates and 15 per cent were having digitalis, judged unnecessary in two-thirds by the authors. Dall (1970) found that three-quarters of patients on continuing digoxin therapy suffered no relapse when the drug was stopped.

Adverse reactions to drugs

Hurwitz and Wade (1969) showed that, of 1268 patients admitted to hospital, 1160 received drugs. 16.2 per cent of these had adverse reactions, of which 80 per cent were of moderate or greater severity. Commonest offenders were digitalis preparations, bronchodilators and ampicillin. Hurwitz (1969) also showed that the incidence of reactions was greater in older patients—the rate in the under 60s was 6.3 per cent while in those aged 60 and over, it was 15.4 per cent. The age trend persisted even when digitalis preparations were excluded. A multicentre study in Britain in 1975 to 1976 (Williamson, in course of publication) showed that 12.5 per cent of patients had drug reactions at the time of admission to a geriatric unit. Learoyd (1972) found that at least 16 per cent of 236 patients admitted to a psychogeriatric service had ill-effects from psychotropic drugs and rapidly improved on their cessation. This author also stated 'at least 20 per cent of admissions to a psychogeriatric unit are directly due to medication'.

It is clear therefore that the problem is immense, and that it will become even more urgent as more and more aged persons confront their doctors for help.

Likewise, it is essential for doctors to have a good understanding of drug use and misuse in old age.

PHARMACOLOGICAL CONSIDERATIONS

Just as infants are highly susceptible to drug effects, so are patients at the other end of life. This is partly the result of true age changes and is a reflection of the increase in biological efficiency from birth to maturity which then falls off with accelerating speed from middle age onwards. Figure 8.1 shows this trend. It also shows the increasing variability which occurs with ageing and which makes a difficult problem even more complex. Some people at the age of 70 show a biological performance superior to that of those 30 or 40 years their junior. For this and other reasons there is a significant alteration in pharmacokinetics with age, the general result being a decrease in tolerance to drug effects (Fig. 8.1).

Changes in body composition have an effect on drug metabolism. There is a significant decrease in lean body mass with increase in metabolically inert tissue with advancing age (Fig. 8.2).

The decrease in metabolically active tissue indicates a reduced dose for many drugs. Certain fat-soluble substances, e.g. many anaesthetic gases, are dissolved to a greater extent in the larger fat deposits of the elderly patient.

Causes of pharmacokinetic changes in old age

This is an extremely complex matter and much uncertainty exists. Much of the evidence is from animal experiments, mainly rats, and important differences exist between this species and man. In addition to the species differences, there is the practical problem of the cost of rearing rats and keeping them alive into old age. The life span of a rat is two to three years. In most studies the oldest rat is 600 days old. It might be argued that much older animals are required to justify extrapolation of results to humans aged 85 to 100 years.

The effect of any drug upon a tissue is dependent upon:

1. its concentration in bioavailable form at the site, and
2. the sensitivity of the tissue to the drug.

The variations in these factors are determined by absorption, distribution, metabolism and excretion of the drug; and these will now be considered in relation to age.

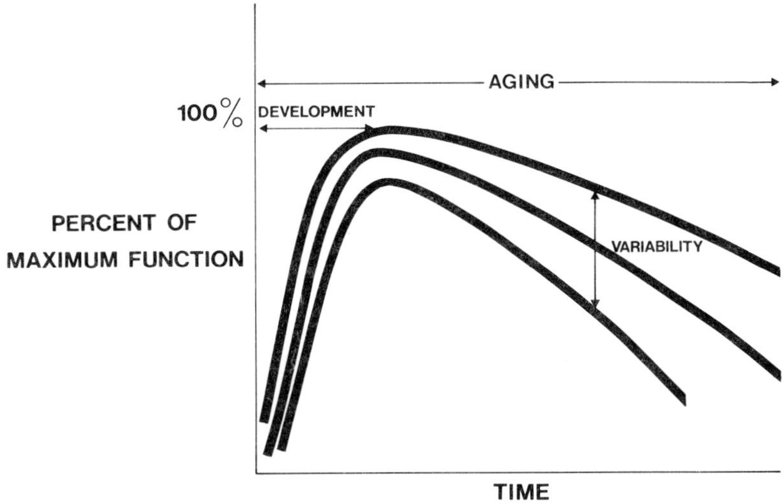

Fig. 8.1 Diagram to show changes in biological efficiency related to age (after Bender, A. D., 1969, *Drug Information Bulletin*, **3**, 153–158)

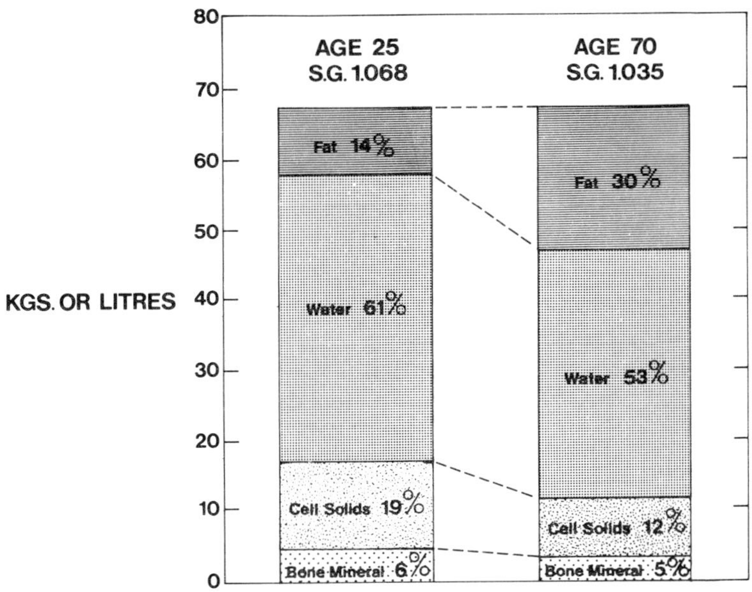

Fig. 8.2 Diagram to show the changes in body composition with increasing age (after Fryer, J. H. 1962, in *Aging Around the World: Biological Aspects of Aging*, ed. Shock, N. W. Columbia University Press)

Absorption of drugs

There is a paucity of information on drug absorption in relation to age. Bender (1968) reviewed age changes which may affect intestinal absorption and concluded that drug absorption is often impaired because of reduced blood flow to the gut; gastric hypochlorhydria (reducing the solubility of some drugs); and reduction in numbers of epithelial cells, leading to a reduced absorptive surface area. Wade (1972) stated that xylose absorption was slower in the aged human; but the original work he cited (Kendall, 1970) was more cautious and concluded (from comparing intravenous and oral tests) that the differences observed in old age were more likely due to renal than intestinal changes. Paracetamol absorption was shown to be reduced in old age (Gwilt et al, 1963) as evidenced by lower blood levels 45 min after ingestion. The issue is complicated by the finding that absorption showed no age deterioration when the preparation was combined with sorbitol. Gorrod (1974) maintained that the findings failed to determine whether absorption was less complete or only delayed.

Concomitantly administered substances affect the absorption of drugs, as in the well-known reduction of tetracycline absorption due to the formation of insoluble complexes if the patient is taking iron, calcium salts or antacids containing aluminium or magnesium. Changes in gut motility likewise influence drug absorption. Any substance which delays or speeds the transit of contents through the small intestine leads to increased or decreased absorption, because of longer or shorter contact with the absorptive surface. Examples are the increased absorption of digoxin when given with propantheline, and the decreased absorption when metaclopromide is given at the same time (Manninen et al, 1973). This experiment was complicated by the finding that only the tablet form of digoxin showed these changes, the liquid form not being affected. These authors make a special plea for avoidance of polypharmacy in patients on digoxin.

Drug distribution in the tissues

Drug distribution in body tissues is influenced by the complex interplay of its chemical and physical properties, the degree of tissue perfusion and the permeability of membranes. Kupferberg and Way (1963) showed increased sensitivity to morphine in 16-day-old rats as compared to 32-day-old animals. Morphine levels in the brains of the 16-day-old rats were two to four times those found in the 32-day-olds. It was concluded that this was due to higher permeability of the immature blood–brain barrier. Bender (1968) postulated that a similar mechanism might account for the increased morphine sensitivity in aged humans. Bromage (1962) showed that a smaller amount of local anaesthetic was required extradurally in elderly subjects to produce a given level of segmental analgesia. This was attributed to increased permeability of nerve membranes and slower elimination due to reduced local perfusion.

Another factor which affects the distribution of many drugs is protein-binding capacity. Many common drugs are bound to a greater or lesser degree to the albumen fraction in plasma. Since only the unbound portion is pharmacologically active, the bioavailability of such substances varies inversely with the degree of binding. The more albumen there is in the plasma, the greater is the binding, and vice versa, so that changes in albumen levels can influence the effect of a drug in this indirect fashion. It is customary to quote the paper of Woodford-Williams et al (1964) as showing that serum albumen levels fall in old age; but these authors were at pains to emphasise that this was not the case in 'normal' ageing, but only in old people who had chronic disorders of various kinds. Hayes, Langman and Short

(1975a) showed a decreased binding of warfarin in elderly patients which they attributed to lowered albumen levels. Warfarin may thus be more available in older patients to produce lower and potentially dangerous prothrombin levels. The same authors demonstrated a marked increase in phenytoin clearance in persons over 65 years, and attributed this to reduced albumen binding.

Where two drugs are given simultaneously, and one has a higher binding capacity than the other, available binding sites may be saturated by the first drug, thus leaving more of the second to exert its effects, which may reach toxic levels. Thus a patient stabilised on tolbutamide may be in danger from hypoglycaemia if a high binding drug such as aspirin or phenylbutazone is added. The danger is greater in older patients with relatively few binding sites, due to hypoalbumenaemia.

Drug metabolism

The main organ concerned in drug metabolism is the liver. The weight of this organ decreases by 28 per cent between the third decade and 70 years and over (Korenchevsky, 1961). Although the liver has a very large reserve capacity, it must be questioned whether the ageing organ can metabolise drugs as speedily and efficiently as in youth.

The metabolic pathway for many drugs is a two-stage process (Williams, 1959) which has been reviewed by Parke (1968) and by LaDu, Mandel and Way (1971). The first stage is usually oxidation, reduction or hydrolysis under the action of microsomal enzymes. This phase has low substrate specificity, so that enzymes induced by the presence of one substance may well actively metabolise another quite unrelated substance. The products of this enzyme reaction are then conjugated with endogenous substances, principally sulphuric or glucuronic acids, and the resulting substance is water soluble and readily excreted.

Animal experiments have shown age-reduction in microsomal enzyme activity. Kato, Chiesara and Frentino (1961) showed that the ability of phenobarbitone to induce enzymes and thus to accelerate meprobamate metabolism was reduced in old rats. The same workers (Kato, Chiesara and Frentino, 1962) showed that liver tissue from old rats metabolised strychnine in vitro more slowly than did liver tissue from young rats. This experiment also showed sex differences in enzyme activity. Using octamethylpyrophoramide, Kato, Takanaka and Omori (1967) showed decreased toxicity in old rats. This can be explained by reduced enzyme activity, the metabolite of the substance being the toxic offender.

It is unwise to relate these animal findings directly to humans, in whom the evidence is much less clear-cut because of the methodological problems involved, especially the large number of variables. Irvine et al (1974) have shown that plasma levels of amylobarbitone are higher 24 h after an oral dose in old subjects than in young persons. They also showed that this is not due to reduced excretion, because they found a correspondingly higher 24-h urinary output of 3′-hydroxyamylobarbitone in younger subjects, this being the principal product of enzyme metabolism of the drug. O'Malley et al (1971) showed a significant increase in the mean plasma half-life of antipyrine and of phenylbutazone in older subjects (+45 and +29 per cent respectively) compared to younger. They also showed marked differences in the half-life of the drug between the two sexes, men apparently being slower metabolisers than women. Some elderly persons were very slow to metabolise both these drugs. The authors postulated that this contributes to the high incidence of adverse reactions in the elderly.

The importance of genetic factors must be mentioned, in so far as they result in a polymorphism in the metabolism of some drugs. This was shown in respect of isoniazid (Knight, Selin and Harris, 1959) and later of sulphamerazine, the same acetylation mechanism being involved. Of more importance to the elderly is the discovery that nitrazepam (Mogadon) is also affected by genetic polymorphism, so that there are fast and slow acetylators. The slow acetylators show significantly higher plasma nitrazepam levels for longer periods than the fast acetylators, and excrete smaller quantities of metabolites of the drug (Karim and Price Evans, 1976). This may help to explain why some elderly persons have adverse effects to relatively small doses of nitrazepam (Grimley Evans and Jarvis, 1972). Nitrazepam has recently also been shown to have more marked and more prolonged undesirable effects in old patients than in younger ones (Castleden et al, 1977). These workers, in a double-blind trial of 10 mg of nitrazepam and placebo showed that at 12 and 36 h elderly subjects felt more drowsy and made more mistakes in psychomotor tests than did younger subjects. This was attributed to increased sensitivity of the ageing brain to the drug, and not to delayed excretion or metabolism, as there was no significant difference in plasma levels or half-lives between old and young subjects. The large-scale use of this hypnotic makes it important to avoid unnecessary hazards in its use.

Drug excretion

The studies of Shock (Davies and Shock, 1950) showed a significant decrease in renal capacity with age. Glomerular filtration rate falls by 46 per cent between youth and old age, renal blood flow by 53 per cent and tubular reabsorption of glucose by similar margins. These workers believe that the decrement is due to reduced numbers of nephrons, those that remain functioning normally.

While the reduced kidney function enables aged subjects to cope adequately with basal demands and those of ordinary living, reserves may be meagre; and any stress such as dehydration or exposure to a nephrotoxic drug precipitates renal failure. Likewise, the capacity of the aged kidney to excrete drugs is compromised. All drugs and their metabolites are filtered by the glomerulus. Those which are highly lipid-soluble are reabsorbed by tubular cells. Drugs may also be actively secreted by tubular cells into the glomerular filtrate. Since all these aspects of renal function are reduced in old age, drugs may attain high plasma levels which may last longer and which increase the dangers of toxic effects. Ewy et al (1969) showed that tritiated digoxin had a plasma half-life of 73 h in men aged 73 to 81 years, compared to 51 h in young subjects. These changes were related to decreased creatinine clearance rates. Caird (1974) confirmed that elderly subjects tended to retain digoxin, and emphasised that plasma urea levels offered a very poor guide to their ability to excrete this drug. Creatinine clearance is a much safer guide; but Baylis et al (1972) maintain that digoxin and creatinine clearances do not have a linear relationship; and they suggest that even a satisfactory creatinine clearance is not an adequate guide. Instead they advocate the use of serial plasma digoxin levels where any doubts exist. The most up-to-date and authoritative statement is from Roberts and Caird (1976) who estimated digoxin clearance, creatinine clearance and steady state plasma digoxin levels on different daily doses of the drug. They found that digoxin and creatinine clearances gave very similar findings and their ratio was close to unity. On a daily dose of 0.25 mg of digoxin, therapeutic plasma levels were obtained provided that creatinine clearance was between 25 and 80 ml/min. Below 25 ml/min of creatinine clearance, this dose resulted in toxic levels. Corresponding figures for a dose of digoxin of 0.125 mg are 5 to 35 ml/min of creatinine clearance, and on a dose of 0.0625 mg/day, therapeutic levels only occur with clearance of less than 10 ml/min and with no danger of toxicity. These authors emphasise that reduction in glomerular filtration rate readily leads to digoxin intoxication as excretion falls. Common causes of sudden reduction in GFR are dehydration, myocardial infarction, and any other cause of reduction of the peripheral circulation.

Similar results occur with antibiotics. Although this may sometimes be advantageous, as in treatment of severe infection by penicillins, the retention of a toxic antibiotic by aged kidneys can be very dangerous (Vartia and Leikola, 1960). Tretracyclines were initially believed to be largely non-toxic in man, but recent reports show them to be potentially highly dangerous, even lethal, in patients with renal impairment. This danger is enhanced by a period of dehydration which is commonly and readily produced in elderly patients (Phillips et al, 1974).

This diminished power to excrete drugs is by far the most important factor in predisposing elderly patients to toxic reactions. Only meticulous care and due regard to lowered starting dose will protect patients. A safe general rule is to start off with a dose about half that for a similar sized young adult, and only gradually increase the dose while watching for toxic effects.

OTHER FACTORS PREDISPOSING TO DRUG HAZARDS IN OLD AGE

The intrinsic factors discussed render old persons unduly vulnerable to drug effects, but other factors may have the same effect.

Multiple drugs

Because old people have multiple illnesses and complaints, they are prone to receive multiple drugs. This is dangerous on account of failing eyesight and hearing, faltering memory and confusion, and unfamiliarity with modern medicine. They are thus less able to comply with the prescriber's instructions. Many studies have shown failure of compliance, and some have been disturbing. Dunnell and Cartwright (1972) found errors of 19 to 36 per cent. Older patients were more likely to have errors of compliance. Stewart and Cluff (1972) reported errors in 25 to 59 per cent of patients, and Libow and Mehl (1970) reported 20 per cent errors in elderly patients. Earnest pleas were made for more complete instructions to patients, with attempts to see that the patient had actually accepted responsibility for controlling medication. Stewart and Cluff (1972) write 'in our society, better instructions are provided when purchasing a new camera or automobile than when the patient receives a life-saving antibiotic or cardiac drug'. It is illogical to insist on vigorous controls in the manufacture, testing and purity of drugs, and then to supply them to the patient in a fashion which results in up to 50 per cent errors. The chain of events from chemical formulation and manufacture to ingestion and tissue effect is only as strong as its weakest link.

Keet (1976) made compliance studies in relation to older patients and found a high correlation of non-compliance with mental impairment. Rather surprisingly, general social and educational level did not seem to influence compliance. Favourable influences were: a strong interest on the part of the physician, and lengthy association between doctor and patient. Sackett et al (1975) found that specific education about hypertension increased awareness of the condition but did not improve compliance in patients on antihypertensive therapy. Keet has conducted experiments using specially designed dispensers which can be loaded with the drugs the patient needs for a period of a week, with each day having one or more compartments. He considered that perhaps three-quarters of the elderly would benefit from such devices and found that errors in compliance were reduced by about 20 per cent by their use. He concluded that cost effectiveness studies were needed to supplement the early investigations. Davidson (1973) investigated the packaging of drugs for old patients and found that the best was a palm-sized transparent container with a screw or snap top. She made a plea for much greater attention to be paid to this matter. She found that 'tear-off' and 'push-through' bubble packings were unsuccessful; although Wade (1972) had suggested that some of the newer forms of presentation might be helpful. It seems obvious that printed instructions in large clear letters should always be used, and that the name of each drug should be spelled out; but often labels are small and the writing is not at all easy to decipher. Wherever possible, a daughter or other relative should be asked to help in supervision. Home helps likewise can fulfil a useful watching role.

Drug interactions

There is now a growing body of evidence on the complex ways in which one drug may interfere with another's action. Problems relating to lowered albumen levels have already been mentioned, as have the effects of drugs which alter intestinal absorption. The problem of enzyme induction by certain drugs has been referred to. This may be important when two drugs are given simultaneously, and each is metabolised by microsomal enzymes. Tricyclic antidepressants and phenothiazines (not an uncommon combination) are both metabolised by the same chemical process. The phenothiazine is a more powerful enzyme-inducer, and if it is stopped less enzyme production will occur, so that the tricyclic substance will be more slowly metabolised with the chance of higher blood levels and toxicity. A patient receiving barbiturate and warfarin may be at risk of warfarin overdosage if the barbiturate is suddenly withdrawn. Some drugs, e.g. chlorcyclizine, glutethimide and phenylbutazone, may inhibit enzymes when they are given 'acutely' and yet they may induce enzyme production when they are given over prolonged periods. Sudden changes in long-standing drug regimes must be carefully considered, e.g. when a patient is admitted to hospital or transfers from one doctor to another. For further information readers are referred to Griffin and D'Arcy (1974).

PRACTICAL ASPECTS OF DRUG THERAPY IN OLD AGE

So far the reader has been subjected to a daunting list of dangers and pitfalls, and may be feeling in despair about ever using drugs in old patients with reasonable safety. It is, however, necessary to keep things in perspective and to remember the enormous benefits which drugs can bestow upon all ages. It is only too easy to take modern drugs for granted and to forget the ghastly toll of infections in previous eras, of the miseries of depressed patients and the revolution in the management of congestive cardiac failure. The fact that powerful drugs are taken for granted no doubt largely explains why they are often over-used.

Special problems

Hypnotics are widely used by old people, especially females. It is generally agreed that barbiturates are undesirable. Most doctors now use a benzodiazepine, usually nitrazepam, which is safe in most respects, although as already mentioned, smaller doses should be tried. Any hypnotic may lead to unsteady gait and the likelihood of falls for the patient who gets up at night. Better management of insomnia by encouraging daytime physical and mental activity may obviate the need for sedatives, which should in all cases only be prescribed for a limited period.

Constipation and faecal stasis are common in old people. The condition may be greatly aggravated by drugs and this may lead to faecal impaction, which is such a common finding in geriatric practice. Caution should be exercised with phenothiazines, tricyclics, and iron preparations; and laxatives should be prescribed if necessary.

Anti-Parkinsonism drugs are potentially dangerous. Dosage should initially be very low with cautious increase and a careful watch for side-effects, which are principally confusion after anticholinergic drugs, and dyskenesia after L-dopa.

Postural hypotension, which may lead to falls and fractures, is commonly caused by tricyclics, phenothiazines, L-dopa and, of course, antihypertensives.

Diuretics, especially the powerful and rapidly acting ones like frusemide, may produce incontinence of which patients (and relatives) should be forewarned. As sudden diuresis in a man with prostatism may produce urinary retention, gentler diuretics should be used, unless the need is for a very powerful drug.

General rules

The first question to be posed is 'Does this patient require drug therapy?' (Hall, 1975) and hence the doctor must define the exact objectives in his management. It is important not to succumb to the temptation simply to 'do something', and to delude oneself that one is being helpful. The current over-use of tranquillisers is an example of this. The intelligent use of a placebo may be appropriate in cases where advice and counselling of patient and relatives is not sufficient. Doctors of previous generations used simple (and totally inert) placebos, while contemporaries prescribe a highly active psychotropic substance with wide effects upon the body systems.

The next requirement is correct diagnosis. While this may be stating the obvious, it is necessary to do so because of the complexity of disease in old age and the fact that few doctors have had special training in geriatric medicine. Common sources of misdiagnosis are toxic confusion, dismissed as dementia; stiffness and locomotor problems dismissed as 'osteoarthritis'; agitation and insomnia due to depression being undiagnosed and treated with hypnotics.

Over-enthusiastic treatment is also fraught with danger. To reduce systolic blood pressure in an 85-year-old is much more likely to do harm than good. Control of diabetes is also a matter for mature judgement, and the relief of symptoms is more important than achieving immaculate control of blood glucose levels.

A golden rule for all prescribing is to use as few drugs as possible in the lowest dosage and in the simplest regime. Doctors should become familiar with a list of valuable drugs, and should not switch to new preparations except for very positive reasons.

Patients should rarely be put on 'repeat prescriptions'. The drug regime should be regularly reviewed. Doctors should be encouraged to prescribe short courses of tranquillisers and then taper the drug till it is ceased. Often this is all that is required.

It is essential to make sure that patients understand the purpose of each drug and the exact dosage and frequency of administration.

REFERENCES

Baylis, E. M., Hall, M. S., Lewis, G. & Marks, V. (1972) Effects of renal function on plasma digoxin levels in elderly ambulant patients in domiciliary practice. *British Medical Journal*, **i**, 338–341.

Bender, A. D. (1968) Effect of age on intestinal absorption: implications for drug absorption in the elderly. *Journal of the American Geriatric Society*, **16**, 1331–1339.

Bromage, P. R. (1962) Exaggerated spread of epidural analgesia in arteriosclerotic patients. Dosage in relation to biological and chronological ageing. *British Medical Journal*, **ii**, 1634–1638.

Caird, F. I. (1974) Metabolism of digoxin in relation to therapy in the elderly. *Gerontologia clinica*, **16**, 68–74.

Castleden, C. M., George, C. F., Marcer, D. & Hallett, C. (1977) Increased sensitivity to nitrazepam in old age. *British Medical Journal*, **i**, 10–12.

Dall, J. L. C. (1970) Maintenance digoxin in elderly patients. *British Medical Journal*, **ii**, 705–706.

Davidson, J. R. (1973) Presentation and packaging of drugs for the elderly. *Journal of Hospital Pharmacy*, **31** (8), 180–184.

Davies, D. F. & Shock, N. W. (1950) Age changes in glomerular filtration rate, effective renal plasma flow and tubular excretory capacity in adult males. *Journal of Clinical Investigation*, **29**, 496–507.

Dunnell, K. & Cartwright, A. (1972) *Medicine Takers, Prescribers and Hoarders*. London and Boston: Routledge and Kegan Paul.

Ewy, G. A., Kapadia, G. G., Yao, L., Lullin, M. & Marcus, F. I. (1969) Digoxin metabolism in the elderly. *Circulation*, **39**, 449–453.

Gibson, I. I. J. M. & O'Hare, M. M. (1968) Prescription of drugs for old people at home. *Gerontologia clinica*, **10**, 271–280.

Gorrod, J. W. (1974) Absorption, metabolism and excretion of drugs in geriatric subjects. *Gerontologia clinica*, **16**, 30–42.

Griffin, J. P. & D'Arcy, P. F. (1974) Drug interactions: I. Sites of interactions. *Prescribers' Journal*, **14**, 7–11.

Grimley Evans, J. & Jarvis, E. H. (1972) Nitrazepam and the elderly. *British Medical Journal*, **iv**, 487.

Gwilt, R. J., Robertson, A., Goldman, L. & Blanchard, A. W. (1963) The absorption characteristics of paracetamol tablets in man. *Journal of Pharmacy and Pharmacology*, **15**, 445–453.

Hall, M. R. P. (1975) Use of drugs in elderly patient [*sic*]. *New York State Journal of Medicine*, **75**, 67–71.

Hayes, M. J., Langman, M. J. S. & Short, A. H. (1975a) Changes in drug metabolism with increasing age: I. Warfarin binding and plasma proteins. *British Journal of Clinical Pharmacology*, **2**, 69–72.

Hayes, M. J., Langman, M. J. S. & Short, A. H. (1975b) Changes in drug metabolism with increasing age: II. Phenytoin clearance and protein binding. *British Journal of Clinical Pharmacology*, **2**, 73–79.

Haynes, R. B. & Sackett, D. C. (1974) An annotated bibliography on the compliance of patients with therapeutic regimens. *Workshop Symposium*, McMaster University Medical Centre.

Hurwitz, N. & Wade, O. L. (1969) Intensive hospital monitoring of adverse reactions to drugs. *British Medical Journal*, **i**, 531–536.

Hurtwitz, N. (1969) Predisposing factors in adverse reaction to drugs. *British Medical Journal*, **i**, 536–539.

Irvine, R. E., Grove, J., Toseland, P. A. & Trounce, J. R. (1974) The effect of age on the hydroxylation of amylobarbitone sodium in man. *British Journal of Clinical Pharmacology*, **1**, 41–43.

Karim, A. K. M. B. & Price Evans, D. A. (1976) Polymorphic acetylation of nitrazepam. *Journal of Medical Genetics*, **13**, 17–19.

Kato, R., Chiesara, E. & Frontino, G. (1961) Induced increase in meprobamate metabolism in rats pretreated with phenobarbital, in relation to age. *Experimentia*, **17**, 520–521.

Kato, R., Chiesara, E. & Frontino, G. (1962) Metabolic differences of strychnine in the rat in relation to sex. *Japanese Journal of Pharmacology*, **12**, 26–33.

Kato, R., Takanaka, A. & Omori, Y. (1967) Factors affecting toxicity and metabolisms of OMPA (octamethylpyrophoramide) in rats. *Japanese Journal of Pharmacology*, **17**, 509–518.

Keet, J. (1976) Failure of the elderly to take medications as prescribed and ways to improve compliance. *Medical Annual*, pp. 208–214. Bristol: John Wright.

Kendall, M. J. (1970) The influence of age on the xylose absorption test. *Gut*, **11**, 498–503.

Knight, R. A., Selin, M. J. & Harris, H. W. (1959) Genetic factors influencing isoniazid blood levels in humans. In *Transactions of the* **18***th Conference on Chemotherapy of Tuberculosis* (St Louis), Veterans Administration, **18**, 52–58.

Korenchevsky, V. (1961) *Physiological and Pathological Ageing*, Basel, New York: S. Karger.

Kupferberg, H. J. & Way, E. L. (1963) Pharmacologic basis for the increased sensitivity of the newborn rat to morphine. *Journal of Pharmacology and Experimental Therapeutics*, **141**, 105–112.

LaDu, B. N., Mandel, H. G. & Way, E. L. (1971) *Fundamentals of Drug Metabolism and Disposition*. Baltimore: Williams and Wilkins Co.

Law, R. & Chalmers, C. (1976) Medicines and elderly people: a general practice survey. *British Medical Journal*, **i**, 565–568.
Learoyd, B. M. (1972) Psychotropic drugs and the elderly patient. *Medical Journal of Australia*, **1**, 1131–1133.
Libow, L. S. & Mehl, B. (1970) Self-administration of medications by patients in hospitals or extended care facilities. *Journal of the American Geriatrics Society*, **18**, 81–85.
Manninen, V., Apajalahti, A., Melin, J. & Karesaja, M. (1973) Altered absorption of digoxin in patients given propantheline and metaclopromide. *Lancet*, **i**, 398–400.
O'Malley, K., Crooks, J., Duke, E. & Stevenson, I. H. (1971) Effect of age and sex on human drug metabolism. *British Medical Journal*, **iii**, 607–609.
Parke, D. V. (1968) *The Biochemistry of Foreign Compounds*. Oxford: Pergamon Press.
Phillips, M. E., Eastwood, J. B., Curtis, J. R., Gower, P. E. & De Wardener, H. E. (1974) Tetracycline poisoning in renal failure. *British Medical Journal*, **ii**, 149–151.
Roberts, M. A. & Caird, F. I. (1976) Steady-state kinetics of digoxin in the elderly. *Age and Ageing*, **5**, 214–223.
Sackett, D. L., Haynes, R. B., Gibson, E. S., Hackett, B. C., Taylor, D. W., Roberts, R. S. & Johnson, A. L. (1975) Randomised clinical trial of strategies for improving medication compliance in primary hypertension. *Lancet*, **i**, 1205–1207.
Shaw, S. M. & Opit, L. J. (1976) Need for supervision in the elderly receiving long term prescribed medication. *British Medical Journal*, **i**, 505–507.
Stewart, R. B. & Cluff, B. L. (1972) A review of medication errors and compliance in ambulant patients. *Clinical Pharmacology and Therapeutics*, **13** (4), 463–468.
Trethowan, W. H. (1975) Pills for personal problems. *British Medical Journal*, **iii**, 749–751.
Wade, O. L. (1972) Drug therapy in the elderly. *Age and Ageing*, **1**, 65–73.
Williams, R. T. (1959) *Detoxication Mechanisms*. London: Chapman and Hall.
Woodford-Williams, E., Alvarez, A. S., Webster, D., Landless, B. & Dixon, M. P. (1964) Serum protein patterns in 'normal' and pathological ageing. *Gerontologia clinica*, **10**, 86–99.
Vartia, K. O. & Leikola, E. (1960) Serum levels of antibiotics in young and old subjects following administration of dihydrostreptomycin and tetracycline. *Journal of Gerontology*, **15**, 392–394.

9. Patterns of delivery of care by departments of geriatric medicine

C. P. Silver

Geriatrics has been defined by the British Geriatrics Society as 'the branch of medicine concerned with the clinical, social, preventive and remedial aspects of disease in the elderly'. In the report of the members of the Royal College of Physicians (1976) geriatrics is defined as 'that branch of general medicine dealing with clinical, social, preventive and remedial factors relevant to maintaining health and independence and to managing illness and disability in old people'. In this definition geriatrics is considered part of general medicine and the description of the preventive and remedial aspects is amplified.

DEPARTMENTS OF GERIATRIC MEDICINE

In 1976 there were 171 departments of geriatric medicine in England and Wales, in charge of some 300 consultants in geriatric medicine (Horrocks, 1976a). There were 222 Health Districts, each serving a population of about one quarter of a million. Some districts were without geriatric services. Under the reorganisation of the National Health Service in 1974, Health Districts were intended to be co-terminous with local authority social service areas, but many hospital geriatric services are not fully aligned to these boundaries. Future trends in geriatric service planning are discussed in a consultative document *Priorities for Health and Personal Social Services in England* (DHSS, 1976a).

Bed provision

In the United Kingdom the Department of Health and Social Security has suggested the following 'norms' of provision of beds and places:

Geriatric beds: England and Wales: 10 beds per 1000 population aged 65 and over
Scotland: 15 beds per 1000 population aged 65 and over.
Acute beds: 2 to 2.5 beds per 1000 population of all ages.
Welfare home places: 25 places per 1000 population aged 65 and over.

These recommendations are calculated to meet a hypothetical average need. Wide differences occur in different districts and actual provision often falls short of the recommended level. In 1974 the average provision in England was 8.57 geriatric beds per 1000 population aged 65 and over (DHSS, 1976a). The recommendations may be too low to meet future needs (British Medical Association, 1976; DHSS, 1976a).

Work of departments of geriatric medicine

Departments of geriatric medicine provide: initial assessment of elderly patients; admission of emergencies; rehabilitation; continuing or long-stay care; and terminal care. In addition they offer planned hospital admission, special collaboration with other hospital departments, and day hospital and outpatient care. They collaborate with general practitioners, community services and welfare homes and undertake preventive measures. They provide information, education and research.

Referral and assessment

Patients come to departments of geriatric medicine from general practitioners or from other hospital departments. Patients referred by social services departments are ordinarily accepted only with the knowledge of the general practitioner; but in the psychogeriatric unit at Nottingham a designated social worker has the same rights of admission as the geriatrician (Morton, 1973). Domiciliary consultations and assessment visits to the home made by the physician in geriatric medicine with the agreement of the general practitioner allow medical and social circumstances to be checked and the need for admission to be determined and ensure efficient use of beds. Visiting by community workers may sometimes be a substitute. The number of assessment visits made varies between different departments, from 2000 in a year (Hospital Advisory Service, 1975) to few or none. Examination in the emergency department or after admission to the ward allows urgent patients to be assessed, while outpatient consultation is satisfactory for other patients.

Progressive patient care

Many departments make use of progressive patient care. Patients are moved from ward to ward according to the different function of each ward, e.g. admission ward, rehabilitation ward, continuing care or long-stay ward. In other departments there are mixed function wards in which long- and short-stay patients are cared for together. The advantage of the former is in concentrating appropriate resources according to ward function; of the latter in diluting heavy with light nursing problems and ensuring a greater feeling of shared responsibility. Farrow, Rablen and Silver (1976) in their study of patients admitted to a geriatric service found that 6 to 8 per cent of male and 8 to 10 per cent of female patients remained in hospital for over one year.

Multi-disciplinary care

Looking after geriatric patients is a team effort. A weekly case conference of those concerned (doctor, remedial therapist, nurse, social worker, home nurse, health visitor) allows an interchange of knowledge and opinions and paves the way to discharge. The patient and relatives attend when necessary. The participants may require additional evidence: mental testing (Hodkinson, 1972) or tests of ability (Silver, 1972); assessment by the occupational therapist, particularly in regard to activities of daily living; visits to the patient's home to see how well the patient manages under field conditions; trial in a discharge flatlet (Howard, 1973); and trial discharge home. Case conferences are additional to and not a substitute for ordinary ward rounds. Communication between staff is made easier by the use of problem-oriented records (Weed, 1969).

Rehabilitation

Rehabilitation takes place either in the ward to which the patient was admitted, or after transfer to a ward deliberately arranged for rehabilitation. Here the patient can be expected to stay for several weeks, until discharge home or elsewhere, or until the decision is made that long-stay care is necessary. Medical treatment, physiotherapy, occupational therapy and speech therapy, good ward morale, art therapy and diversional activities all increase the chance of improvement and discharge.

Continuing or long-stay care

Unlike some other countries (Brocklehurst, 1975) Great Britain has set itself against providing long-stay hospital or residential care on an enormous scale—rather the aim is to provide adequate housing, satisfactory domiciliary services and, where necessary, warden-controlled accommodation. However, some patients do require long-stay hospital accommodation. Rainey, Russell and Silver (1975) found that in the East London borough of Tower Hamlets 91 patients (0.41 per cent of the population aged 65 and over) had been in hospital for over one year in beds for the physically ill and 70 per cent of these were demented, i.e. the commonest reason for occupation of a long-stay geriatric bed was a combination of physical and mental disorder. This inevitably means that continuing care wards are less active and cheerful than wards where patients are leaving to go home. Visitors to continuing care wards often complain that patients are 'sitting staring at the walls'. In part this is due not to apathy and loss of a sense of purpose, as it was in former days in the workhouse, but to mental changes. The atmosphere can be improved by great efforts of the staff, a patients' association, encouraging relatives to take part in the care of patients and the provision of a relatives' corner in the ward, relatives' conferences, the efforts of volunteers, and home visits for the weekend or afternoon. No continuing care ward should be without some kind of regular review in case medical or social circumstances change. Besides a general review, investigation of specific matters such as dental state (Payne et al, 1973) and vision (Fenton, Arnold and Wilkins, 1975), are important.

A valuable booklet on *Improving Geriatric Care in Hospital* dealing with factors affecting the quality of the patient's life and preservation of human dignity has been published jointly by the British Geriatrics Society and the Royal College of Nursing (1975).

Planned hospital admissions

Arrangements designed to help the elderly patient remain within the community include DeLargy's 'six-weeks-in-and-out' scheme of regular hospital re-admission (DeLargy, 1957), a revolving door principle of admission, often less elaborately undertaken than when originally described; variations of this scheme (Griffiths and Cosin, 1976); the five day hospital and home for the weekend (Parnell and Naylor, 1973); and the admission of ill or severely disabled patients to relieve relatives going on holiday.

COLLABORATION WITH OTHER DEPARTMENTS

The psychogeriatric assessment unit

Many sick old people suffer from combinations of physical and mental disease. The psychogeriatric assessment unit is the meeting place where geriatrician and psychiatrist can jointly assess such patients. It serves as the centre of a combined geriatric and psychogeriatric service. The geriatrician also has a role in the care of physical illness in mental hospitals (Hall, Lloyd and MacLennan, 1974). The situation is further discussed in Chapter 10.

The geriatric orthopaedic unit

Elderly patients occupy a considerable number of orthopaedic beds (Table 9.1). Orthopaedic surgeons have found that collaboration with the geriatrician in jointly run units can be useful (Devas, 1970). The initial treatment is undertaken by the orthopaedic surgeon, usually with the involvement of the geriatrician at an early stage; later rehabilitation and discharge is mainly in the hands of the geriatrician. The joint approach takes into account the considerable proportion of elderly patients presenting with fractures as a complication of physical ill health (e.g. bone disease and arthritis, cerebrovascular disease, anaemia) or whose fracture is the most arresting event in a downward course due to dementia. It also takes account of the multiple pathology, complications occurring after the injury and the slower rehabilitation of older patients. As Devas points out, an operation can be successful only if the patient returns to independence; and this aim is more easily achieved in a combined unit.

The stroke unit

It has been suggested that stroke units are well placed in the geriatric service (Isaacs, 1976; Kennedy, 1976). Isaacs found that one-third of the patients referred to a stroke unit in Glasgow were under the age of 65, 40 per cent were aged 65 to 74 years and rather less than one-third were aged 75 and over. A stroke unit brings together patients already occupying hospital beds, and brings effective treatment to bear upon their problems.

Amputees

Another example of collaboration is the care of elderly amputees (Clarke-Williams, 1973).

The day hospital

The day hospital is an important feature of geriatric care. Brocklehurst (1970) described day hospitals available up to 1970. In 1975 the number of regular day patient attendances was in excess of one million (DHSS, 1976c). The provision recommended is two places per 1000 population aged 65 and over. Day hospitals provide medical and nursing care for elderly patients who do not require hospital admission yet who need more than outpatient consultation. They allow the patient to be examined at leisure, to be cared for over a day, while nursing, physiotherapy and occupational therapy are carried out without hurry. Since the patient stays for a meal they also assist with nutrition. They differ from local authority day centres in providing specific therapy and skilled supervision rather than social facilities only. Day centres provide a useful outlet for patients whose main reason for attendance at the day hospital has become social. In St Matthew's Hospital, London, a social club and day centre is run by the local authority in the same hospital building as the day hospital serving day patients and inpatients (Silver, 1970). Psychogeriatric day hospitals are an important aspect of psychiatric care of the elderly.

Quality of geriatric services

Although geriatrics is the fastest growing of all specialties, and although enormous improvements have been made in the service, the position throughout the country is not satisfactory. The Hospital (now Health) Advisory Service has almost finished surveying all geriatric departments on a Domesday Book principle. Successive reports draw a disturbing picture of gross inadequacies in many geriatric departments and, while highlighting many areas where good standards of work prevail and interesting innovations are being tried, yet paint overall gloomy pictures of poor facilities, inadequate staffing and numerous deficiencies which must be remedied. The inverse care law (Hart, 1971) often applies, districts most in need having the worst services. The Department of Health has recommended that at least 50 per cent of geriatric beds should be in the district hospital, but nearly one-fifth of all Health Districts have no designated geriatric beds in general hospitals (DHSS, 1976a). In general, it may be said that services are inadequate when beds are not provided in general hospitals.

RELATIONSHIP BETWEEN GERIATRICS AND GENERAL MEDICINE

Geriatrics and general medicine overlap. Difficulties may arise in districts where the relationship between geriatric medicine and general medicine is neither defined nor agreed. Patients aged 65 and over occupy some 50 per cent of all hospital beds. Table 9.1 shows

Table 9.1 Hospital beds occupied by elderly patients. Estimated average numbers of beds used daily, England and Wales

		General hospital beds (departments)				
Age	All	General medical	General surgical	Trauma and orthopaedic	Geriatric	Psychiatric hospital beds
65–74	35 088	7 571	5 498	2 653	11 743	22 843
75+	56 640	5 987	4 126	4 081	37 474	23 806
All ages	188 171	27 717	25 156	17 862	53 659	100 888

Sources. General hospital beds: Hospital Inpatient Enquiry, 1973
Psychiatric hospital beds: Beds occupied on 31st December 1973 (DHSS).

the average number of general medical, general surgical, and trauma and orthopaedic beds occupied daily compared with the number of geriatric and psychiatric beds. The length of stay of patients in the first of these categories is short but rises with age. In 1973 the mean duration of stay was 14.0 days for all general medical patients compared with 20.8 days for patients aged 75 and over. In 1975 the average duration of stay for geriatric patients was 93.8 days; in general medical wards there was a 'throughput' of 24.3 cases per year on average, compared with 3.6 cases per year in departments of geriatric medicine.

Table 9.2 shows the number of discharges and deaths in general medical and geriatric departments in the United Kingdom in 1973. These are equivalent to the number of

Table 9.2 Estimated total discharges and deaths from general medical and geriatric departments, 1973, England and Wales

Age	General medical	Geriatric
65–74	160 580	51 660
75+	105 260	140 230
All ages	724 460	200 430

Source: Hospital Inpatient Enquiry, 1973.

admissions. There were more than three times as many admissions to general medical beds as to geriatric beds of patients aged 65 to 74, but of patients aged 75 and over a majority were admitted to geriatric beds.

DEFINITIONS OF THE 'GERIATRIC PATIENT'

Defining geriatrics is fairly straightforward; defining the 'geriatric patient' in any sense other than purely administrative, that is a patient attending a department of geriatric medicine, is impossible. Indeed, the British Geriatrics Society condemns the term 'geriatric patient'. It could be said that everyone believes that he knows who is a 'geriatric patient' but no one can define one satisfactorily.

The geriatric patient defined by disability

From a practical point of view, e.g. the award of extra salary to nursing staff working in geriatric departments, the definition of a geriatric patient is one who is looked after by a consultant geriatrician in a bed designated as geriatric by the Department of Health. But this is no help in drawing any precise distinction between medical and geriatric patients. In practice there is none. There are only elderly patients, showing a complete spectrum of disease and disability, as do patients in other age groups. If they remain ill for long enough they develop the characteristics common to all sick old people. Eventually they present with combinations of physical, mental and social difficulties. Patients usually looked after by a geriatric department present these combinations in good measure. They are defined, therefore, by disability. Often the decision to call a patient 'geriatric' is made by the referring general practitioner, working in accordance with local custom.

Outcome of care of elderly patients in 'medical' and 'geriatric' units

In the London borough of Tower Hamlets, where the care of old people is shared between geriatric and medical units, there were in 1974, 636 admissions of patients aged 75 and over to the geriatric service and 919 to general medical beds. One-third of the former and one-quarter of the latter died in hospital. Sixty-one per cent of the 'geriatric' patients and 67 per cent of the 'medical' spent less than 28 days in hospital. Fifty-one patients from the medical wards were transferred to geriatric beds, and of these, 11 were subsequently discharged home. Some 60 to 65 general medical beds were continuously occupied by patients aged 75 and over. Many patients were admitted just as quickly to the geriatric as to the medical wards. The differences in mortality and outcome between the two groups may be because more disabled patients went to the geriatric department.

The 'geriatric patient' defined by age

Much less commonly 'geriatric patients' are defined by age. In some areas all patients over a certain age who do not require specialised services are accepted by the geriatrician. The age selected should distinguish between two groups of patients with different characteristics. Evans, Hodkinson and Mezey (1971) considered that geriatrics should be defined as the comprehensive care of the sick aged 75 and over, the service being organised by a geriatrician whose role embraces both hospital and community care. O'Brien, Joshi and Warren (1973) described the arrangement in Oldham where all patients aged 65 and over are accepted by the geriatric service. In one year there were 1661 admissions of patients aged 65 and over to their geriatric service and only 191 to general medical beds in the same district. In Burnley the age limit is 70 (Hajela, 1976) and in Hull, 75 (Horrocks, 1976b).

Other approaches

Other proposals for rationalising the hospital care of the elderly include a measure of fusion of medical and geriatric services, and, more radically, the virtual abolition of geriatrics.

Joint medical and geriatric teams

Many patients and their relatives look with alarm on the prospect of admission to geriatric wards. However, admitting all patients aged 75 and over to the geriatric department does not necessarily imply complete segregation. Grimley Evans (1976) has described the arrangements in Newcastle where combined teams look after all admissions including the elderly, in jointly run wards. Each team comprises a consultant in general medicine, a consultant in geriatric and general medicine and a specialist physician.

Abolish geriatrics?

Leonard (1976) suggested that geriatrics as a separate specialty should be largely abandoned, except perhaps in a few centres retained for teaching and research. His suggestion was made to solve the difficulty in attracting medical staff to departments of geriatric medicine. His argument can be refuted on several grounds. When joint staffing of general medical and geriatric departments is accepted, many staffing difficulties will disappear. Hospital admission is only one aspect of the work of departments of geriatric medicine. Those who are deeply involved with the elderly look beyond the hospital and take a wider view than the general physician of their responsibility not only for the individual patient, but for the development of services that will be needed in the future. To make advances, great problems of logistics and education must be overcome; and to abolish the specialty of geriatrics would be to remove the driving force needed. Progress in geriatrics has come from influences outside medicine, from the policies of the DHSS and from the work of specialist geriatricians, and not, with rare exceptions, from general physicians. This is not gainsaying the clinical advances over the whole field of medicine which have benefited elderly patients.

POLICIES OF DEPARTMENTS OF GERIATRIC MEDICINE

The measurement of health and personal social services in the elderly is complex (Jackson and Himatsingani, 1973). Accounts of successful policies and practices in departments of geriatric medicine are often descriptive and have been prepared without reference to comparable data either before the arrangement under review was set up or in a neighbouring district.

The 'high turnover' department

Three broad patterns of working can be discerned in departments of geriatric medicine. First is the 'high turnover' department, for example the department at Northwick Park Hospital, Harrow, with a turnover of 6.16 admissions/bed per year discussed by Hodkinson and Jefferys (1972). They admitted most of their patients on the day on which they were referred by the general practitioner. They regarded the support of the general practitioner as crucial and did not visit patients at home. They secured more numerous discharges and these took place earlier than in comparable units. They felt that high turnover dealt with problems more effectively, although they were sometimes forced to accept less than full therapeutic response. The real choice might not be between early and late discharge but between discharge and no discharge at all. Good staffing and a substantial number of beds within the district hospital were available. Critics of their approach may feel that success cannot be entirely measured by turnover. Accepting turnover as the main criterion could mean missing the most difficult patients with which only geriatricians deal, the so-called 'hard-core' (Isaacs, Livingstone and Neville, 1972).

The 'comprehensive' department

The second kind of department concentrates on a comprehensive geriatric service, with many community ramifications and more emphasis on the less urgently ill, on the lines sketched by Woodford-Williams (1967). However, the high turnover and the comprehensive approaches are not incompatible, provided sufficient resources are available to provide both kinds of service.

O'Brien et al (1973) in Oldham base their method of working on six points:

1. Total medical care with responsibility for all medical emergencies in the 'pensionable' age group and with many beds in the district general hospital;
2. Assessment at home of non-urgent cases.
3. High turnover (6.1 admissions/bed per year) and no waiting list.
4. A wide choice of help for the general practitioner.
5. Early consultation with colleagues in other specialties, particularly orthopaedic and accident and emergency departments.
6. Free interchange of appropriate cases between psychiatric and geriatric departments.

The 'low turnover' department

The third type of department, the 'low turnover' department, is based on custodial attitudes. 'Low turnover' departments act usually as a back-up service for general medical wards, with comparatively few admissions directly from the community. The Hospital Advisory Service, with unrivalled opportunity for comparing geriatric departments, describes difficulties over admission, 'blocked beds', problems of 'disposal' and difficulties over discharge after long waits before admission as the invariable accompaniment of a 'low turnover'. Insufficient resources with inadequate staffing and lack of beds in the district hospital are the usual explanation of low turnover, but in some unsatisfactory departments, where the number of beds available is higher per head of population than in 'high turnover' departments, the differences in performances have to be attributed to differences in ways of working.

THE GENERAL PRACTITIONER, COMMUNITY SERVICE AND WELFARE HOMES

In the Report of the Chief Medical Officer for 1974 (DHSS, 1976b) it was estimated that in a representative district with a population of 250 000 there are 35 000 people aged 65 and over. Of 925 000 general practitioner consultations in the course of a year, 200 000 are with the elderly. Elliott and Stevenson (1973) considered that the general practitioner looked to the geriatrician for specialised advice about the care of the elderly, through the agencies of domiciliary consultations, hospital outpatient clinics, clinics in health centres and admission to hospital on a long- or short-stay basis.

Table 9.3 shows the use of the principal community services in 1975. The figures represent a heavy, increasing, and inextricably mixed load on health and social services.

Adequate community services make care at home more practical. It is essential for the geriatric department to tap these resources. The formation of primary health care teams in which home nurse, health visitor and social worker are attached to practices improves co-operation with the hospital geriatric service. After discharge from the geriatric service, those patients who are regarded as 'at risk' receive surveillance from health visitors, community nurses and social workers who report both to the general practitioners and to the geriatric service.

Table 9.3 Use of Community Health and Social Services by persons over 65 (England).

	Thousands	
	1970	1975
Persons treated by home nurses	530.5	929.2
Persons having contact with health visitors	369.3	548.9
Persons receiving chiropody treatment	828.6	1235.4
Persons receiving home help	373.3	533.3
Persons receiving meals at home from local authorities (Meals on Wheels)	24.6	53.3
Persons receiving meals at home from voluntary agencies (Meals on Wheels)	85.1	111.8
Number of households containing a person aged 65 and over receiving aids and adaptations	—	174.3

Source: Department of Health and Social Security, *Annual Report, for 1975.*

Support for residential homes

Many welfare home residents are admitted without any medical assessment, since the grounds for admission are 'social'. Lowther and McLeod (1974) examining residents within a week of admission, considered that 36 per cent should have been admitted to hospital rather than to a home. There is a place for support of residential homes by departments of geriatric medicine in advising general practitioners and in the education of staff.

CONCLUSION

This chapter can be summarised by considering the choices open to a newly appointed consultant in a district where geriatric services need development. His aim will be to control a department closely associated with other hospital departments playing a key role in the care of the elderly in the community. There will be a number of decisions to be taken, some of which are influenced by circumstances which he cannot alter and all of which depend on the resources he can muster. The social character and resources of the district in terms of housing, hospital services, community services including welfare homes, voluntary homes and organisations, must be accepted, though over a period of time he may have the opportunity of influencing them. It will be worth considering whether local authority social service boundaries and geriatric service boundaries can be made coterminous. He will have to decide whether to aim at a high turnover service, perhaps accepting some limitation on the completeness of the service, or whether resources allow a more comprehensive service. He may find a low turnover service which he can only alter by concentrating on certain parts of the service. He must also choose between a disability-defined and an age-defined service. He may start with the former and make his way toward the latter. Rather than building up a separate and self-sufficient department he may want a more broadly based department, regarding the geriatric organisation as the spine controlled by the specialist geriatricians, with help from consultants in general medicine. Finally, knowing that the department has much to offer, he will expect help from general practitioners and community services.

REFERENCES

British Geriatrics Society and Royal College of Nursing (1975) *Improving Geriatric Care in Hospital.* London: Royal College of Nursing.

British Medical Association (1976) *Services for the Elderly.* London: British Medical Association.

Brocklehurst, J. C. (1970) *The Geriatric Day Hospital*. King Edward's Hospital Fund for London.
Brocklehurst, J. C. (1975) *Geriatric Care in Advanced Societies*, ed. Brocklehurst, J. C. Lancaster: MTP.
Clarke-Williams, M. J. (1973) In *Textbook of Geriatric Medicine*, ed. Brocklehurst, J. C., pp. 524–527. London: Churchill Livingstone.
DeLargy, J. (1957) Six weeks in: six weeks out. *Lancet*, **i**, 418–419.
Department of Health and Social Security (1976a) *Priorities for Health and Personal Social Services in England*. London: HMSO.
Department of Health and Social Security (1976b) *On the State of the Public Health. Annual Report of the Chief Medical Officer for the year 1974*. London: HMSO.
Department of Health and Social Security (1976c) *Annual Report 1975*. London: HMSO.
Devas, M. B. (1970) Treatment of patients with fractures near the hip. *Modern Geriatrics*, **1**, 45–56.
Elliott, A. E. & Stevenson, J. S. K. (1973) Geriatric care in general practice. *Journal of the Royal College of General Practitioners*, **23**, 615–625.
Evans, G. J., Hodkinson, H. M. & Mezey, A. G. (1971) The elderly sick, who looks after them? *Lancet*, **ii**, 539–541.
Evans, J. G. (1976) Personal communication.
Farrow, S. C., Rablen, M. R. & Silver, C. P. (1976) Geriatric admissions in East London 1962–1972. *Age and Ageing*, **5**, 49–55.
Fenton, P. J., Arnold, R. C. & Wilkins, P. S. W. (1975) Evaluation of vision in slow-stream wards. *Age and Ageing*, **4**, 43–48.
Griffiths, R. A. & Cosin, L. Z. (1976) The floating bed. *Lancet*, **i**, 684–685.
Hajela, V. P. (1976) Personal communication.
Hall, M. R. P., Lloyd, C. M. & MacLennan, W. J. (1974) The role of the geriatrician in mental hospitals. *Age and Ageing*, **3**, 36–42.
Hart, J. T. (1971) The inverse care law. *Lancet*, **i**, 405–412.
Hodkinson, H. M. & Jefferys, P. M. (1972) Making hospital geriatrics work. *British Medical Journal*, **iv**, 536–539.
Hodkinson, H. M. (1972) Evaluation of a mental test score for assessment of mental impairment in the elderly. *Age and Ageing*, **1**, 233–238.
Horrocks, P. (1976a) In *Doctors and Old Age*, ed. Leeming, J. T., pp. 23–28. Mitcham: British Geriatrics Society.
Horrocks, P. (1976b) Personal Communication.
Hospital Advisory Service (1975) *Annual Report*. London: HMSO.
Howard, R. J. (1973) Rehabilitation flat. *Health and Social Services Journal*, **83**, 1192–1193.
Isaacs, B. (1976) The place of a stroke unit in geriatric medicine. *Physiotherapy*, **62**, 152–154.
Isaacs, B., Livingstone, M. & Neville, Y. (1972) *Survival of the Unfittest*. London: Routledge and Kegan Paul.
Jackson, R. R. P. & Himatsingani, C. (1973) In *Needs of the Elderly*. ed. Canvin, R. W. & Pearson, N. G., pp. 11–25. Exeter: University of Exeter.
Kennedy, B. F. (1976) The stroke unit—a physiotherapist's view. *Physiotherapy*, **62**, 154–155.
Leonard, J. C. (1976) Can geriatrics survive? *British Medical Journal*, **ii**, 1335–1336.
Lowther, C. P. & McLeod, H. M. (1974) Admission to a welfare home. *Health Bulletin*, **32**, 14–18.
Morton, E. V. B. (1973) The team approach. *Symposia on Geriatric Medicine*, **2**, 45–55.
O'Brien, T. D., Joshi, D. M. & Warren, E. W. (1973) No apology for geriatrics. *British Medical Journal*, **iv**, 277–280.
Parnell, J. W. & Naylor, R. (1973) *Home for the Weekend—Back on Monday*. London: Queen's Institute of District Nursing.
Payne, P. E. C., Evans, D. J., Stafford, G. D. & Bates, J. F. (1973) Dental survey of geriatric patients in hospitals in the Cardiff area. *Age and Ageing*, **2**, 39–45.
Rainey, C. G. E., Russell, W. F. & Silver, C. P. (1975) Long-stay patients in the London borough of Tower Hamlets. *Age and Ageing*, **4**, 247–254.
Royal College of Physicians (1976) Care of the elderly. Report of the Standing Committee of Members. *Journal of the Royal College of Physicians*, **10**, 276–284.
Silver, C. P. (1970) A jointly sponsored geriatric social club and day hospital. *Gerontologia clinica*, **12**, 235–240.
Silver, C. P. (1972) Simple methods of testing ability in geriatric patients. *Gerontologia clinica*, **14**, 110–112.
Weed, L. L. (1969) *Medical Records, Medical Education and Patient Care*. Cleveland, Ohio: Press of Case Western Reserve University
Woodford-Williams, E. (1967) The function and structure of a geriatric department. *Gerontologia clinica*, **9**, 199–205.

10. Conflict and collaboration between geriatric medicine and psychiatry

Colin Godber

The reader will need no reminder of the extent to which frailty in the elderly has overtaken the resources of our medical and social services, threatening to engulf them over the next couple of decades. This chapter will concern itself with one of the most troublesome points of leakage in the system, the 'psychogeriatric' problem.

OVERLAP BETWEEN GERIATRIC MEDICINE AND PSYCHIATRY

A number of epidemiological studies (e.g. Williamson et al, 1964; Kay, Beamish and Roth, 1964) have demonstrated the extent and overlap of physical and psychiatric morbidity in the elderly, and the interaction of the two has been reviewed recently by Anderson and Davidson (1975). The Newcastle workers have also shown the heavy demand on hospital and residential services of those with organic brain syndromes (Kay et al, 1970) and the frequency of psychiatric morbidity amongst those occupying general medical beds (Bergmann and Eastham, 1974). Both types of morbidity reach their highest prevalence in the over-75s whose vulnerability is compounded by the frequency with which bereavement and geographical separation from family and friends has enforced a solitary existence. It is, of course, this age group in which the most dramatic expansion has been taking place, with projections for the UK of a further 40 per cent rise by the end of the century.

Unfortunately the wider appreciation of these facts and of the disadvantage at which the services for the elderly are already working has come at a time when health care planning has shifted from 'ideals' to 'priorities', with the British transition rougher than most because of the enforced cessation of 'growth' in public expenditure. It is, perhaps, fortunate that we have advanced further than many countries in the evolution of geriatric medicine, a specialty which has shown its potential in working out priorities and improving efficiency in its sector of the care of the elderly. Geriatricians have not always been afforded the room for manoeuvre necessary for such achievements, often as a result of the ambivalence (e.g. Leonard, 1976) of their general hospital colleagues. A further handicap has been the variability of resources and support amongst coproviders of institutional care for old people, i.e. psychiatrists and departments of social service.

This chapter will be particularly concerned with the response from psychiatry, and with ways in which effective partnership may enable geriatrics to increase its effectiveness and its impact on the care of old people. Because of the difficulty in drawing comparisons between services in different countries, with their variable distribution between public and private provision, between welfare and health, and between primary and specialist care, consideration will be directed at the situation and prospects in the United Kingdom. It is hoped, however, that the models discussed will be of relevance to those working with the elderly under different systems.

THE 'PSYCHOGERIATRIC' PATIENT AND THE HOSPITAL SERVICES

The author will deliberately avoid defining the 'psychogeriatric patient'. For most people other than psychogeriatricians, who are also indefinable, they are 'geriatric' patients (i.e. disabled old people who seem to be in the way) with the added characteristic of being or appearing to be confused. Many of these identified by Kay et al (1964, 1970) as occupying places in hospital did so in long-stay beds on account of the nursing requirements of advanced dementia itself. For others the nursing needs were for physical disabilities, with dementia as a coincidental or complicating factor. In both of these groups the lack of someone outside hospital to provide the nursing care is usually an important factor in their hospitalisation, as was demonstrated in the earlier Newcastle study (Kay et al, 1964) by the high proportion of severely demented patients found to be still in the community. This social factor is also relevant to many psychogeriatric patients in acute hospital beds, where admission for an illness normally manageable at home may have been triggered by lack of necessary domiciliary supervision.

When the facilities for the care of old people are over-subscribed, the label of morbidity becomes an important passport to such care. In the case of the 'psychogeriatric' patient the labels of 'mental impairment', 'physical disability' and 'need for residential supervision' may coincide. This makes for a blurring of responsibility, which often results in the patient gravitating to whichever service is most accessible at the time when the need is most pressing.

THE CURING SPECIALTIES

Since intercurrent ailments are a frequent source of crises in the 'psychogeriatric' patient, the acute hospital services, with their traditional availability of beds for patients presenting as bona fide medical and surgical emergencies, often admit patients for whose needs their skills are only tangentially appropriate. This has tended to harden the 'psychogeriatric' stigma. What makes these patients particularly unpopular with 'acute specialties' is that admission often marks a point of final breakdown of a long-standing precarious existence at home. This may mean that an alternative placement has to be found before discharge. A family which has coped with decreasing enthusiasm with a confused parent may find that acute hospital admission for intercurrent illness provides the only, and perhaps a long-awaited, chance to opt out of their responsibility. In such cases, the awareness of these potential problems for discharge by the hospital staff is often belated, and all too rarely do those who were involved in the patient's care before his admission make adequate provision for his discharge. Such situations frequently extend the spell in hospital, out of all proportion to the medical or surgical needs underlying the admission. The other side of this coin is that many patients in acute confusional states who were coping well before admission, and who could be expected to do so after discharge, are thought erroneously to share the gloomy outlook described previously. This may also result in unnecessary delays in rehabilitation and discharge.

THE 'CARING' SPECIALTIES

Considerable progress has been made towards the problem of aligning the hospital services to the needs and disability patterns of elderly people with the development of the specialty of geriatric medicine. The effective geriatrician bases management (and particularly the decision as to whether or not to admit to hospital) on a thorough preliminary assessment of the patient's social, mental and physical status. This principle permits rational use of resources and facilitates early planning for future needs. The geriatrician's potential is most fully realised when he has created, or has been given, enough room for manoeuvre to provide a sizeable part of the acute care in hospital for the elderly. In this way problem patients present directly rather than appearing as the bedraggled rejects of the general physician. Even here, however, the problem of gravitation persists, and geriatricians have found themselves increasingly expected to absorb the 'psychogeriatric' problem too. This is where the conflict with psychiatry tends to arise.

Psychiatry responded much later than medicine to the organisational problems of its chronically disabled elderly, the majority of whom are suffering from dementia. The more effective management of the functional psychoses over the last 20 years emptied thousands of mental hospital beds, and made it less noticeable that many were filling up with elderly dements. The escalation of this trend, and pressure from the DHSS towards bed reduction in the mental hospitals, created amongst psychiatrists in the last decade increasing anxiety about the psychogeriatric problem. The reaction to this anxiety was very varied, with the Freudian mechanism of 'denial' all too common. The lessons of geriatric medicine show that no effective service can derive from the vacuum of a purely custodial pattern of care, and that someone has got to go out and face the problem.

MODELS OF PSYCHOGERIATRIC SERVICE

Ways will now be discussed in which the initiative has been taken by or on behalf of psychiatry to cope directly with those elderly people whose main morbidity label is 'psychiatric'.

'Compleat geriatricians'

When the 'psychogeriatric' problem was tackled positively, the initiative usually came from departments of geriatric medicine, though the Department of Health and Social Security (DHSS) has encouraged and facilitated collaboration between the specialties. Geriatric physicians carry a considerable caseload of demented patients whose physical needs justify a medical pattern of supervision and nursing. Many geriatric physicians also see the provision of acute hospital care as an important component of their services to the frail elderly, and encounter in this way a number of the 'psychogeriatric' patients portrayed earlier as inappropriate clients of the specialist medical unit. In other cases, the lack of coherent psychiatric activity at the 'non-medical' end of the 'psychogeriatric' field led to the geriatricians taking over that responsibility as well.

Examples of such physician-run dementia services are described by Lodge (1976) and by Portsmouth (1974). In these two instances the geriatrician, with the agreement or at the invitation of the psychiatrist, took over the clinical administration of a number of wards in the mental hospital; these have been run in conjunction with his own geriatric medical service and with variable involvement of psychiatrists. This left the geriatric physician with a broader control of the hospital services for the elderly. This permitted a more unified admission policy, and removed the problem of demarcation for admission between 'geriatric' and 'psychogeriatric' patients. Lodge (1976) extended this facility by setting up a short-stay psychogeriatric assessment unit in conjunction with the long-stay area.

A more extreme example is the psychogeriatric unit in Middlesborough described by Prinsley (1973), a geriatric physician. This acute 'psychogeriatric' unit catered for a wide range of psychiatric illness in old people, many of whom had no 'medical' label at the time of presentation. There was minimal cross consultation with psychiatrists. Patients suitable for transfer to long-stay psychiatric care generally found their way to geriatric (medical) long-stay wards. The high turnover through this unit implied that it was meeting a local need by providing speedy admission, which was not available through orthodox channels. This certainly was a commendable attempt to fill a gap in a local service, but it extended the geriatrician well beyond the field of his own expertise and training. It can hardly be put forward as a model for psychogeriatric provision for the future.

THE JOINT PSYCHOGERIATRIC ASSESSMENT UNIT

The question of the limits of expertise, in medical and nursing staff, was raised by the work of Kidd (1962). In a study of groups of elderly people admitted to geriatric and psychiatric units he identified a significant proportion who might be designated as 'misplaced' in terms of the appropriateness of their major clinical problem to the unit in which they found themselves. Patients in the 'wrong' unit seemed to fare worse in terms of mortality and length of stay in hospital. Subsequent studies (Mezey, Hodkinson and Evans, 1968; Copeland et al, 1975) failed to replicate these findings and cast doubt on the validity of Kidd's data and interpretation. Andrews et al (1972) regarded misplacement as a manifestation of inadequate services, with patients in crisis going wherever a bed was available, even if this was clinically inappropriate. This factor of urgency might also explain the tendency to higher mortality. Nevertheless Kidd's work played its part in the evolution of a model of collaboration between geriatric medicine and psychiatry in the care of the elderly mentally infirm which was to be based on the Joint Psychogeriatric Assessment Unit (PGAU).

The joint PGAU became the cornerstone of DHSS policy (1970, 1972) on psychogeriatric care. A number of these units had already sprung up in the 1960s. Such units, comprising 15 to 30 beds, were ideally sited in or adjacent to the Geriatric Assessment Unit on the campus of the District General Hospital (DGH). They were run jointly by a consultant in geriatric medicine and a psychiatrist who headed a multidisciplinary team of nursing staff, remedial therapists and a social worker. The psychiatrist would not necessarily specialise in the care of the elderly, though one psychiatrist in each district might concentrate on this role and would thus be sucked into greater involvement in the field. Patients were admitted to the PGAU by either the geriatrician or the psychiatrist, preferably after preliminary assessment at home. Full assessment and clinical investigation in the unit, appropriate treatment and rehabilitation, and the outcome of enquiries made by the social worker then permitted a joint decision to be reached as to the appropriate placement for the patient.

The clientele of this unit predominantly comprised patients with dementia in whom thorough assessment revealed complicating but treatable disorders and gave guidance on future placement. Elderly people suffering from functional illness continued to be served by general psychiatric units. The DHSS plans were not clear as to the management of the many patients in whom dementia and functional illness coexisted. Patients with confusional states which had been triggered by acute physical illness were catered for by the acute medical services under the aegis of the general, or of the geriatric, physicians. The recommendations for demented patients with acute exacerbations of their confusion due to identified physical illness were not clear. An unknown factor was the proportion of demented patients identified by the geriatric and psychiatric services who needed to pass through the joint PGAU.

The PGAU as a sorting-station

There was much to recommend the use of the PGAU as a sorting-station for patients who were likely to require long-term care in mental hospital beds, and for a small proportion of those with both dementia and major physical disability who might ultimately reach long-stay geriatric beds. There were also patients with apparent need for residential care, for whom fuller assessment and rehabilitation might pave the way to such care or even forestall it. In addition was the need presented by crises and transient deterioration so common among demented patients, for which short periods of hospital care were necessary. With this potentially very large caseload the bed requirements for the PGAU anticipated by the DHSS (10–20 beds per 250 000 general population) necessitated a rapid turnover of patients.

Blockage in the PGAU

This points to a particular vulnerability of the PGAU in terms of its capacity for discharge of patients. Apart from the normal problems of negotiating patients' discharge to their own homes or to a residential home the PGAU also had to place a significant proportion of its patients in long-stay geriatric (medical) and psychiatric beds. If there was a hold-up in the transfer of patients to the geriatric area the unit increasingly took on the characteristics of a long-stay geriatric ward. If there were such difficulties in the geriatric department, these were likely to be problems in admission of patients to geriatric short-stay beds, which in turn led to misplacement of 'medical geriatric' cases into the joint unit, who added further to the queue waiting for long-stay geriatric beds. The equivalent pattern occurred when the blockage was in the psychiatric part of the service and even more seriously when there was blockage in both. Similar problems occurred when there were delays in the placement of patients in residential homes.

It takes only a small number of patients blocking beds in this way to start the vicious circle which is the downfall of any short-stay unit in the 'geriatric' field. With fewer beds in circulation turnover falls; with fewer discharges fewer admissions are possible and emergencies cease to be catered for. Waiting lists develop, resulting in frayed tolerance amongst relatives and others caring for patients (e.g. in residential homes). This produces more refusal to accept patients back after treatment, increasing the blockage further. Really urgent cases are diverted as 'social admissions' to acute medical or psychiatric beds, with all the loss of initiative and delay in rehabilitation that is implied in this.

This tale of woe is not, of course, the inevitable fate of the joint PGAU, but it is liable to be fulfilled if such a unit is seen as a panacea for the 'psychogeriatric' problem. The PGAU can function only if the two contributing services, geriatric medicine and psychiatry, function well in their own right. Their long-stay commitments should not exceed their resources, and their use of the joint unit should adhere to a firm operational policy. This is frequently not appreciated by those planning such units.

A successful joint service

In West Cornwall, which is frequently used as a model of the DHSS plan in effective action (Donovan, Williams and Wilson, 1971) the problem of maintaining a thriving geriatric medical service in the absence of an equivalent focus in the psychiatric service led the geriatrician to tripartite planning with his psychiatric and local authority colleagues of facilities needed to cope with the looming problem of the elderly mentally infirm. From this emerged a joint PGAU and day hospital which were based in the same hospital as the acute geriatric unit. At the same time the long-stay geriatric and psychiatric services were rationalised and two residential homes specialising in the care of the mentally infirm were established. This collaboration extended to the drawing-up of operational policies aimed at minimising the bottlenecks and barriers referred to earlier. The clinicians also played an important role in the two homes, whose residents were assessed in the joint unit prior to admission. An effective 'psychogeriatric' service resulted, despite the large geographical spread of the catchment area and the high proportion of elderly people within it. One interesting later by-product was the creation within the psychiatric service of a consultant post with special responsibility for the elderly. Because of the size of the caseload, however, this 'geriatric psychiatrist' can only extend activities into the functional illness of the elderly to a limited extent.

'THE GERIATRIC PSYCHIATRIST'

The models discussed hitherto have represented attempts to coax psychiatrists into the application of certain well-established principles of 'geriatrics' to the management of mentally infirm elderly patients. There were, however, a number of pioneers in psychiatry who needed no such coaxing and who set up their own 'comprehensive' psychiatric services for old people (Robinson, 1965; Whitehead, 1965). This trend has increased markedly over the last few years, stimulated partly by the enthusiasm of its participants (Arie, 1972; Pitt, 1974) and partly by the concern of many local health authorities to plug what they see as a major gap in their services. This trend has not been officially endorsed by the DHSS, which, though hinting at changes, has not yet contradicted its 1972 policy statement on 'Services for Mental Illness Related to Old Age' which attempts to separate the services for organic and functional illness in the elderly. It does seem likely, however, that the DHSS and the Royal College of Psychiatrists will find themselves carried along with the new tide, some of the implications of which will now be considered.

The raison d'être of the geriatric psychiatrist is two-fold. In the first place the mixture of functional and organic aetiology, the atypical presentation and the complicating physical and social factors of mental illness in old age warrant specialisation in the same way as in medicine. Similarly, just as the organisational aspects of the department of geriatric medicine frequently outweigh technical skills in their contribution to the success of the service, so the focusing of responsibility for 'psychogeriatric' care in one specialist offers the opportunity of a more efficient use of the resources available to the service, and of better liaison with other agencies.

A COMPREHENSIVE PSYCHIATRIC SERVICE FOR THE ELDERLY

In a 'comprehensive psychiatric service for the elderly', the aim is usually that, given sufficient quantity and quality of resources, the geriatric psychiatrist will cater for the bulk of psychiatric illness in the over 65s in his district. He will obviously accept that a number of people, especially in the younger strata of this age range, may be served as well or better by the general psychiatric unit. Conversely the needs of patients with presenile dementia will usually tally better with his own service. The management of the chronic psychotic patient who has grown old in the mental hospital is usually left to the general psychiatrist, unless there are supervening problems of dementia or frailty. The justification is that this 'graduate' clientele has already achieved a pattern of care in the mental hospital which will not be changed by age alone and that such a large extra inpatient commitment would add to the handicaps of a specialist whose caseload is largely located in the community.

Priorities

By including in his unit both functional and organic psychiatric disorder the geriatric psychiatrist has to balance the provision of his service between three factors: the demand for treatment of reversible disorders; support through crises in fluctuating chronic disorders; and longer term support of heavily disabled patients. Most geriatric psychiatrists place a high priority on the use of short-term care as a way of tackling the first two categories, on the basis that this will reduce the overall level of disability in the community and will help those supporting the chronically disabled to continue to do so. Since delays in meeting identified treatment needs and crises can only be harmful, the capacity to admit emergencies without delay is crucial. All of this implies careful screening of new referrals, usually at home.

The range of services provided by geriatric psychiatrists varies considerably. Excellent accounts are given by Arie (1972) and by Pitt (1974). In the present author's service which is probably fairly representative, the catchment area comprises just over 200 000 people of whom about 28 000 are aged 65 and over. There are 125 beds (which is more than the DHSS 'norm'), but very little day care. A service is offered along the lines outlined above, catering for about 95 per cent of psychiatric referrals in patients aged 65 and over. During the three years that the service has operated, the referral rate of new cases has risen from 400 to just under 550 a year, and admissions from 300 to 550 (100 of these in the first year and 150 in the last were planned relief admissions). The number of beds used for short stay is 50, of which two-fifths are occupied by patients with functional illness, just under one-sixth by planned relief admissions, and the rest by acute and chronic organic brain syndromes. All patients are assessed before admission, and extensive follow-up is carried out by community-based nurses and medical staff. The latter are particularly involved with those patients in residential homes. The increasing referral rate has brought forward greater numbers of patients with functional illness and more 'younger' (65–75 year old) people. Some tendency has been noted to earlier referral of those with dementia.

Because of local difficulty in obtaining acute geriatric admissions, general practitioners refer a number of patients with clear physical illness, some of whom are admitted. The ability to admit emergencies means that there are fewer major problems in discharging patients, though negotiation of discharge before admission remains an important aspect of the initial assessment. As a result of this, and of support in residential homes and the programme of intermittent relief care, the flow of patients into long-stay beds can be controlled and predicted, and there is no backlog in the short-stay area. Because of the slower tempo of the geriatric department it is not possible at present to operate a joint admission unit. Nevertheless liaison is close and a considerable volume of cross-referral of patients takes place. The geriatric senior registrars are seconded to the psychogeriatric unit for part of their training.

Advantages of the geriatric psychiatrist

There seem to be a number of advantages in a full-time geriatric psychiatrist. In the first place this permits rationalisation of the use of facilities on the basis of a heavy commitment in the community. The case for defining the service by the age of the patient rather than by the type of illness is strongly supported by the variable and often bizarre presentation of functional illness in the elderly, the indication from local hospital turnover figures that we are picking up a 'new clientele' in that sphere, and the gratifying results of treatment. As the nucleus of inpatients with functional illness increases it becomes possible to admit younger patients who might earlier have baulked at entering a 'psychogeriatric unit', with benefit to the morale and standards of the unit. Morale in the long-stay wards also improves. The service is seen by general practitioners as a therapeutic as well as a caring one. More than a little enthusiasm for the subject is engendered in trainees, particularly from psychiatry, who pass through the unit. Finally liaison is improved with geriatric physicians, social services, the residential homes, voluntary services and the housing department.

COLLABORATION BETWEEN GERIATRIC PSYCHIATRIST AND GERIATRIC PHYSICIAN

Although the 'geriatric psychiatry' model makes responsibilities more clear-cut at the psychiatric end of 'psychogeriatrics', it does not necessarily resolve conflict at the medical end. It provides, as a counterpart to the geriatric physician, a specialist who shares similarities in outlook and skills, and with whom there is mutual interest in collaboration.

In the DHSS plans the joint PGAU was to have been the focal point of collaboration, and the main channel for the psychogeriatric service. The 'geriatric psychiatrist' admits many patients who do not require the attention of his colleague in geriatric medicine. His medical expertise enables him to cope with many aspects of physical illness. Arie and Dunn (1973) found that the joint inpatient care requirements in their service, which deal with a catchment area comprising approximately 25 000 elderly, can be met by a four-bedded unit based in one of the geriatric medical admission wards. Both consultants have the right to admit to this unit, and to discharge or transfer to the appropriate bed once the need for joint care has passed. With both services able to admit patients as quickly as necessary the problems of blockage discussed above do not arise. The emphasis in this unit therefore is on bringing together both specialists in the care of patients with mixed problems, with acceptance by the nursing staff of this hybrid clientele. Patients with less overlap of medical and psychiatric problems are treated in the appropriate unit and the other specialist's advice is sought on management. This flexibility is enhanced by the readiness of each consultant to accept admissions to his ward on the recommendation of his colleague after a home assessment.

In the Royal Victoria Hospital in Edinburgh (Robinson, 1975) both services have clinics, day hospitals and short-stay beds on the same site only a few yards apart. Joint consultation is practised at each level of care. One quarter of the patients seen at home by each consultant are brought subsequently to the clinic for 'joint assessment'. Cross-consultation occurs in the day hospitals and the admission wards, and the consultants attend each other's ward conferences. The nursing staff seek each other's advice, and transfer of patients from one unit to the other is very easy, and thus seldom necessary. There is no formal 'joint care unit', as in the service of Dunn and Arie. One reason for this is that most of the nursing staff in both the geriatric and psychiatric wards are general-trained, so that 'joint nursing' would not greatly enhance the range of skills. This service demonstrates that, where the facilities encourage it, a considerable amount of clinical interaction between geriatric psychiatry and medicine occurs. The process is facilitated by the matching catchment areas and by the capacity of each service to meet demands.

DUAL SPECIALISATION

In future it would seem desirable to plan our services on the basis of dual specialisation, i.e. geriatric medicine and geriatric psychiatry. This bilateral commitment does not automatically provide the answer; large gaps may remain between the two services through which many of the most difficult patients fall. Some consideration will therefore be given to these remaining sources of difficulty and ways in which they may be overcome.

Catchment areas

It is difficult for two services to link their activities if their catchment area boundaries are not co-terminous. The different development of geriatric and psychiatric services may require a geriatric department to liaise with three or four psychiatric services, whose ways of dealing with the care of the elderly may vary considerably. The tendency to geographical sectorisation of psychiatric services, to meet district rather than traditional mental hospital boundaries, goes some way to reducing this problem. In the creation of posts for geriatric psychiatrists it is therefore particularly important to secure the same catchment areas as the geriatric physician. Common catchment areas also facilitate liaison with social service departments, general practitioners and other hospital specialties.

Difference in tempo

Another barrier to liaison between departments of geriatric medicine and psychiatry is difference in tempo, with one providing an on-demand service, while the other admits only from a waiting list. The problem of the ailing service may be due to lack of beds, as compared for instance with accepted DHSS norms (1971, 1972) low though these may seem. If this is the case the proportion of beds used for long stay must be strictly rationed. One method is to designate some of these for programmes of regular intermittent relief, thus squeezing three to four patients into a bed. Another is to use part of this long-stay area to create a ward for acute or rehabilitation short-stay care. This measure is seldom attractive to geriatric physicians, who naturally wish to restrict such care to the DGH, but is not impossible if patients are selected carefully and is not without benefit to the morale and standards of the long-stay hospital itself.

In many cases the problem of slow turnover is not related to actual bed shortage but to blockage of short-stay beds by patients awaiting transfer to long-stay wards or elsewhere. This requires review of the admission policy and the home assessment procedure, or redeployment of staff to improve the effectiveness of rehabilitation in the short-stay area. Often more than one of these factors is present. They have to be unravelled if departments are to work more closely and if the acute work of the ailing service is not to have to be done rather randomly by its opposite number and by the general medical wards. Real bed shortages need to be made up; in the case of geriatric medicine this may involve a transfer of beds and staff from the general medical empire, a step which seldom appeals to the general physicians. In other instances there may need to be a shift between the two 'geriatric' departments, where the desire to work more closely together may provide the motivation for such generosity on the part of the better endowed service, even though its own resources may already fall short of the norms mentioned above. While recommending such ad hoc methods for getting services working the author would echo the sentiments of

Jolley and Arie (1976) that one must never forget that the provision of a rationed service, the demand on such a service and the need in the community at large are very different quantities.

A JOINT DEPARTMENT OF GERIATRIC MEDICINE AND PSYCHIATRY

These considerations highlight the degree of give-and-take that is necessary between geriatric psychiatry and geriatric medicine if a coherent hospital service for the elderly is to emerge. Ironically it is often the confused physically disabled patient, the patient most in need of a 'geriatric' service, who is failed by the two specialties, either because each thinks the other should accept responsibility, or because the need for care is too urgent and devolves on the general medical unit. One way of maximising joint consultation and care is for the two specialties to merge into one administrative unit. Some shifting of resources and alteration of operational policies would be necessary to ensure that patients' needs were met with equal speed and thoroughness at both the medical and the psychiatric end of the scale. This would apply to hospital and community care and would end the situation of one part of the service being worse than the other. The easiest way to shift beds from one service to the other is to allow long-stay beds in the better-endowed section to be filled by patients with the other type of disability, or to turn over some short-stay beds to joint care.

Boundaries with other specialties

Another aspect of reallocation of resources is determination of boundaries with general psychiatry and general medicine respectively. The geriatric psychiatrist might be able to provide a service for all patients aged 65 and over, but a higher age boundary between general medicine and geriatric medicine is necessary. The geriatric department would be responsible for the provision of emergency care for patients in its age group on the understanding that physicians would not expect high priority for transfer to the geriatric service of their patients whose rehabilitation and discharge were difficult.

Advantages of joint care

The merging of the two services would greatly extend the proportion of outpatients, day patients, short- and long-stay inpatients who received joint care. Joint inpatient care may bring together nursing staff of medical and psychiatric backgrounds. It may alleviate the difficulty of mixing confused and non-confused patients in long-stay wards. Referral by general practitioners is simplified. Consultants of either specialty have admission rights throughout the service, and might use joint outpatient assessment on a scale comparable to Robinson's (1975) service. Joint supervision at every level of care facilitates training and cross-fertilisation of ideas among medical and nursing staff. It also makes for easier relationships between the 'geriatric' service and the 'community hospitals'. Relations between the two geriatric specialties and other hospital disciplines will change. A 'cogwheel' division of geriatrics might emerge, which should seek representation on the district medical committee structure. The resulting improved standing and influence of 'geriatricians' vis-à-vis their hospital and general practitioner colleagues will benefit recruitment of staff and allocation of resources. A strong unified hospital 'geriatric' department will be in a better position to influence attitudes to the care of the elderly of social service and housing departments, which should increase their readiness to accept advice on the employment of their own resources and the planning of future provision. More coherent support to the general practitioner stimulates his cooperation in preventive geriatrics.

CONCLUSION

The conflicts described in this chapter are similar to those in other fields of social and health care where provision has not kept pace with demand, let alone need, and where multiple disability makes it uncertain where responsibility lies. The specialty of geriatric medicine has shown how much can be achieved clinically in the care of old people, and equally encouraging results have emerged from similar specialisation within psychiatry. Psychiatrists must apply what has been learnt in the geriatric field about the effective use of resources. Where geriatric specialists have managed to keep their houses in order and to make a significant impact on their local services it has been by careful preliminary assessment of patients, maximum turnover through treatment areas, and rationing of longer-term supportive care. The maintenance of such a service is easier if emergencies are coped with rather than diverted to a less appropriate quarter. This 'misplacement by default' has been most frequent with the psychogeriatric patient. It may be hoped that dual specialisation in the care of the elderly will ensure that few patients needing 'geriatric' care reach other specialists by default. If provision for this middle ground is secured, referral rates will reflect more closely the real need in the community.

The overlap between geriatric psychiatry and geriatric medicine and the value of clinical interaction make separate administration of their services superfluous. It is counterproductive for the two specialties to have different levels of performance. The creation of joint departments should facilitate the work and improve communication. The joint department constitutes a more powerful base for influencing local provision for the elderly, while at the same time making 'geriatricians' accountable for the costly resources at their disposal.

REFERENCES

Anderson, W. Ferguson & Davidson, R. (1975) In *Modern Perspectives in the Psychiatry of Old Age*, ed. Howells, J. G., Ch. 5. London: Churchill Livingstone.

Andrews, J., Bardon, D., Gander, D., Gibson, K. B., Mallett, B. C. & Robinson, K. V. (1972) Planning of psychogeriatric care: a report of a joint working party of geriatric physicians and psychiatrists. *Gerontologia clinica*, **14**, 100–109.

Arie, T. D. H. (1972) Aspects of the Goodmayes service. In *Approaches to Action*, ed. McLachlan, G., Ch. 2. London: OUP.

Arie, T. & Dunn, T. (1973) A 'do-it-yourself' psychiatric–geriatric joint patient unit. *Lancet*, **ii**, 1313–1316.

Bergmann, K. & Eastham, E. J. (1974) Psychogeriatric ascertainment and assessment for treatment in an acute medical ward setting. *Age and Ageing*, **3**, 174–188.

Copeland, J. R. M., Kelleher, M. J., Kellett, J. M., Harron, G., Cowan, D. W. & Gourlay, A. J. (1975) Evaluation of a psychogeriatric service: the distinction between psychogeriatric and geriatric patients. *British Journal of Psychiatry*, **126**, 21–29.

Department of Health and Social Security (1970) Psychogeriatric assessment unit. *Circular HM(70) 11*. London: DHSS.

Department of Health and Social Security (1971) *D.S.* **329/71**.

Department of Health and Social Security (1972) Services for mental illness related to old age. *Circular HM*(**72**)**71**. London: DHSS.

Donovan, J. F., Williams, I. E. I. & Wilson, T. D. (1971) A fully integrated psychogeriatric service. In *Recent Developments in Psychogeriatrics*, ed. Kay, D. W. K. & Walk, A., Ch. 10. London: RMPA.

Jolley, D. J. & Arie, T. (1976) Psychiatric services for the elderly: how many beds? *British Journal of Psychiatry*, **129**, 418–423.

Kay, D. W. K., Beamish, P. & Roth, M. (1964) Old age mental disorders in Newcastle upon Tyne. *British Journal of Psychiatry*, **110,** 146–158.

Kay, D. W. K., Bergmann, K., McKechnie, M., Foster, E. M. & Roth, M. (1970) Mental Illness and Hospital usage in the elderly: a random sample followed up. *Comprehensive Psychiatry*, **11,** 26–35.

Kidd, C. B. (1962) Misplacement of the elderly in hospital: a study of patients admitted to geriatric and mental hospitals. *British Medical Journal*, **ii,** 1491–1495.

Leonard, J. C. (1976) Can geriatrics survive ? *British Medical Journal*, **i,** 1335–1336.

Lodge, B. R. W. (1976) A dementia service. Paper read at BGS meeting at Keele University, May 1976. To be published in *Gerontology*.

Mezey, A. C., Hodkinson, H. M. & Evans, G. J. (1968) The elderly in the wrong unit. *British Medical Journal*, **iii,** 16–18.

Pitt, Brice (1974) *Psychogeriatrics*. London: Churchill Livingstone.

Prinsley, D. M. (1973) Psychogeriatric ward for mentally disturbed elderly patients. *British Medical Journal*, **iv,** 169–170.

Portsmouth, O. H. D. (1974) Psychogeriatrics: a design for care of mentally ill older people. *Geriatrics*, **29,** 142–149.

Robinson, R. A. (1965) A psychiatric geriatric unit. In *Pychiatric Disorders in the Aged*. W. P. A. Symposium, pp. 186–205. Geigy.

Robinson, R. A. (1975) In *Nuffield Provincial Hospital Trust Seminar of Psychiatry of Old Age* (unpublished).

Whitehead, A. (1965) A comprehensive psychogeriatric service. *Lancet*, **ii,** 583–586.

Williamson, J., Stokoe, I. H., Gray, S., Fisher, M., Smith, A., McGhee, A. & Stephenson, E. (1964) Old people at home: their unreported needs. *Lancet*, **i,** 1117–1120.

11. The early detection and prevention of disease in the elderly

Sir Ferguson Anderson

Geriatric medicine can be defined as a branch of general medicine dealing with the health and with the clinical, preventive, remedial and social aspects of illness in older people. Health is mentioned first since preventive aspects of geriatric medicine are perhaps the most important part of the subject. In future, physicians will be expected to keep people healthy, rather than to treat them when they are ill. With the conquest of infectious disease, the main problems to be solved in medicine are the early detection of chronic disease and the prevention of further disability. Most physicians who deal with elderly people find that these patients report to them at a relatively late stage in their illness. More could have been done if the individual had sought medical attention at an earlier stage.

EXPERIENCE OF PREVENTION AND EARLY DETECTION

The Rutherglen experiment (Anderson and Cowan, 1955) was started in a public health clinic in an endeavour to examine apparently healthy older people, to integrate medical treatment with social and environmental services for the elderly, and to reduce demand on hospital beds in geriatric departments by avoiding unnecessary admissions. Information about available services was provided. The patients were referred by their general practitioners and were examined by a consultant physician specialising in geriatric medicine. From the experience at Rutherglen it was found that there were three lines of attack against disease in old people: to aim at retaining physical health as age advanced; to maintain mental health; and to preserve social standing and circumstances.

The following principles developed from this work:

1. The general practitioner should control early ascertainment of illness and should be kept informed of results. He should remain in sole charge of his patient and of any treatment ordered.
2. When the older person is seen by the physician in geriatric medicine, no hint or expression should be used to convey that the specialist's diagnosis or treatment is better than that of the general practitioner, and no steps should be taken to weaken the bond between general practitioner and patient.
3. Immediate admission to a geriatric unit or a general hospital should be possible for assessment, diagnosis and treatment.

Unreported illness

Williamson (1966) used the term 'unreported illness' to refer to his finding that although old people felt unwell, might have pain and find difficulty in leading an ordinary life, they did not bring to the notice of their medical advisers such symptoms as painful feet, difficulty in walking, trouble with micturition, anaemia and dementia. The symptoms were attributed by the patient to ageing and not to disease. This tendency might be due to the fatalism of old people or their relatives, or their fear of being put away somewhere, admitted to hospital or institution and never allowed home; or it may occur because many older people are mentally impaired and cannot seek medical advice.

Williamson et al (1964) showed, in a random sample of elderly men and women taken from the lists of three general practitioners, that the average number of disabilities (defined as lesions causing the person to be less well than he should be) in males was 3.26, of which an average of 1.8 were not known to the general practitioner; and in females 3.42 and 2.03 respectively. Just over half of the disabilities detected in the survey were previously unknown to the general practitioner. Thus, older people on occasion could not tell when they were unwell, so that disease was not detected at an early stage. There is an 'iceberg' of unreported illness among older people in the community.

Detection

Keeping older people in their own homes for as long as they desire and are able involves training all who work with the elderly—nurses, medical students, doctors, paramedical staff and social workers—in the special ways in which disease presents in older people, and in the methods of detecting illness at an early stage. These are the principles of preventive geriatric medicine. Writing on the problem of unreported illness in general practice and the methods needed for detection, Currie (1975) stated that 'old age should be anticipated and prophylactic geriatric care should be given in middle life'.

ASSESSMENT OF HEALTH

A number of studies have been conducted of health and disability of samples of old people in the community.

Surveys of disability

In a study of randomly selected people aged 65 and over in the small Scottish town of Kilsyth, Andrews, Cowan and Anderson (1971) demonstrated a marked increase in morbidity with age. Many of the conditions discovered were remediable. The main medical problems found were cardiac failure, anaemia, urinary symptoms, deafness and failing sight.

Williams et al (1972) classified 297 people aged 75 years and over who were examined in general practice, into three categories of health. The first group showed no sign of incapacitating illness, had normal mobility, were able to do housework and shopping and were in a cheerful mental state. The second suffered from some state of ill-health with which they were able to cope, even though their movements were restricted. In the third category were people suffering from incapacitating illness or mental deterioration which had made them bedfast and unable to cook. One hundred and seventy-seven (60 per cent) of the subjects were in Category 1, 108 (36 per cent) were in Category 2, and 12 (4 per cent) were in Category 3. Seventy-five per cent of those seen could be helped. Every person gained something by participating in the examination even if only the psychological benefit of being told that he was in good health.

Ruikka (1971) found in Finland that the old, more than any other group, suffered from hidden illness or disease, with very few symptoms. In Ontario, Canada, 600 people aged

79 and over were surveyed by Schwenger (1971) using public health nurses. Many unmet needs were discovered.

A randomly selected group of 808 people aged 65 and over living at home, were studied by Akhtar et al (1973). Disability was defined as inability to exist at home without help, and dependence as a further degree of impairment of self care. The prevalence of disability increased from 12 per cent in those aged 65 to 69, to over 80 per cent in those aged 85 and over. In 48 per cent of the 227 disabled subjects a neurological disorder contributed to disability; 22 per cent had a functional psychiatric disorder, 38 per cent a cardiorespiratory diagnosis, 24 per cent joint disease, 16 per cent obesity, 11 per cent visual impairment and 3 per cent persistent incontinence. In women aged 75 years and over with neurological disorder the two great problems were non-vascular dementia and disturbance of balance. The prevalence of 'dependence' was 2 per cent of those under the age of 85 and 25 per cent of those aged 85 and over. Of the 27 dependent subjects, 93 per cent had a neurological disorder, 77 per cent were demented and 33 per cent were persistently incontinent.

Non-cooperation

In an attempt to assess the state of health of those who did not cooperate in the survey Akhtar (1972) showed that the physical and mental health of those who refused to take part were very similar to those who agreed. Milne, Maule and Williamson (1971) also found that those who refused and those who agreed to participate in their survey resembled each other in respect of many medical characteristics. Pike (1969) reported relatively little unmet need among people who failed to attend a screening examination. Elderly people who fail to participate in surveys do not seem to be a high risk group.

Diet and nutrition

While nutritional disease is rare in the elderly (DHSS, 1972; Macleod, Judge and Caird, 1974a, b, 1975), many old people have an inadequate intake. In the Kilsyth study, 26 per cent of subjects aged 65 years and over needed dietary guidance (Andrews et al, 1971). Of 116 patients in a general practice who were aged 75 years and over and who lived alone, 23 had less than one cooked meal a day (Williams, 1974). An inadequate diet was found more commonly in women, in the 80 to 90 age group and in the widowed. Hodkinson et al (1973) showed that elderly women with biopsy-proven osteomalacia had the same dietary vitamin D or calcium intake as elderly women without osteomalacia, but had significantly less exposure to sunlight, largely because they were confined to the house. Housebound old people are at the greatest disadvantage because they lack exposure to sunlight and often have very low dietary intakes. This subject is discussed in Chapter 5.

Mental health

In older people failing mental reserve occurs at a time of increasing physical frailty associated with traumatic experiences such as bereavement, compulsory retirement and falling income.

Anxiety and depression. At the Rutherglen consultative clinic, anxiety and depression, which because of their severity merited attention, were observed in 13 per cent of men and 18 per cent of women in good physical health, and in 31 per cent of men and 38 per cent of women with physical disease. The incidence of emotional disturbance did not increase with age, while the proportion due to physical ill health declined with age. There were usually multiple causes, of which the commonest were physical disease, adverse home environment, which included the state of living alone, bereavement, personal ill-health and ill-health of a relative. Enforced retirement was a commoner problem in men than in women. Financial difficulty by itself was rarely a cause of anxiety or depression, but was often a secondary factor. This confirmed the finding of Sheldon (1948). Parental neglect by all the children in one family was not commonly found.

Numerous studies (Stenbäck, 1975) have revealed the high incidence of depression in older people in the community and the close association between depression and physical disease. Busse (1969) stated that social and economic levels affected the frequency of depressive episodes. The low income group of elderly subjects had a considerably greater incidence of depression than higher income subjects. Social deprivation was of frequent occurrence in the Kilsyth survey (Andrews et al, 1971) and was usually part of a complex network of illness which involved body or mind.

Social isolation enhances the chances of admission to a mental hospital, especially among the elderly. Two-thirds of the beds in mental hospitals occupied by people aged 65 years and over are taken up by single, widowed or divorced people. Macmillan (1960) has stated that when an old person lives in isolation, either psychological because of lack of interest, antagonism, self-pity or resentment on the part of relatives, or actual because of solitude, deterioration sets in. Mayer-Gross, Slater and Roth (1960) state that isolation created by vicissitudes such as bereavement, is often aggravated by physical infirmity and declining vision and hearing.

Intellectual loss. Busse (1965) noted that with ageing, intellectual skills were lost to a significant degree in the poorly educated, whose occupation placed them in a lower socioeconomic class. The intellectual loss was greatest in those individuals who could least afford such a decline.

PREVENTIVE MEASURES

The following measures are important in the maintenance of the health of elderly people in their own homes: early diagnostic health examination; preretirement training; re-employment bureaux; mutual aid schemes; retired employees' associations; hobbies and craft centres; all-day clubs and lunch clubs; telephone reassurance; friendly visiting; sheltered housing; homes for the physically and mentally frail; TV, radio programmes; news-sheets; continuing education for the retired.

EARLY DIAGNOSTIC HEALTH EXAMINATION

Since 1948 many surveys of unmet need in the elderly have been undertaken (British Medical Association, 1976). A system must be devised which combines the traditional self-reporting of symptoms with unobtrusive surveillance. Such a system is best implemented through the primary health care team. The initiative must be taken in finding those conditions in elderly people which could be improved with treatment. In the United Kingdom the Family Practitioner Committee can provide a list of all patients in a general practice who are aged 65 and over. The BMA Report warns against purposeless visiting which might worry an otherwise independent and healthy individual and convert him into a 'patient'. Opportunities must be created for the elderly to express to a sympathetic member of the team any matters relating to their physical, social or mental well-being. One method of doing this is to arrange for health visitors attached to the general practitioner to visit persons aged 70 years and over, the age at which the prevalence of disability becomes high (Akhtar et al, 1973) and at which dietary surveillance is important (Exton-Smith and Stanton, 1965).

Role of the health visitor

A nurse routinely visiting old people in their own homes should obtain job satisfaction. If the people visited are almost all fit and require no assistance it is difficult to sustain the interest of the nurse. In the age group 65 to 69, some 10 per cent of men and 13 per cent of women would benefit from a visit by a health visitor; whereas in the 70 to 74 age group 26 per cent of the men and 59 per cent of the women would benefit. This percentage rises further with increasing age. A health visitor is acceptable to the elderly and does not precipitate the danger of changing a client to a patient, as the unexpected and uninvited call of a doctor might do.

The health visitor reports her findings to the general practitioner. In many cases the services needed can be arranged by the health visitor with the general practitioner's knowledge and approval, while the doctor may wish to examine a small number himself.

Performance of the health visitor

When old people were examined separately by a health visitor, a geriatrician and a psychiatrist, Williamson, Lowther and Gray (1966) showed that there was a good correlation of findings between health visitors and doctors in the detection of physical but not of psychiatric illness. Powell and Crombie (1974) demonstrated that a health visitor, using a questionnaire, could detect nearly all the physical, mental and social illness to be found in older people living in their own homes, but could not make an exact diagnosis of psychiatric illness.

The value of early detection

In a study from general practice reported by Barber and Wallis (1976) patients were referred for assessment to the health visitor by other members of the practice team with whom they were already in contact. The value of this screening method lay in the discovery of a large number of minor disabilities which, had they been left untreated, might have resulted in severe handicap. For each patient there was a mean of 4.8 medicosocial problems, one unmet need and 2.3 unknown symptoms. This confirmed a statement by Thomas (1968). The patients assessed in Barber and Wallis's study were all previously known to the practice doctor and to the health visitor. However, as problems and disabilities become multiple with advancing years, it is increasingly difficult for one person to remain aware of them all.

Williams et al (1972) considered that even if it was impossible to treat effectively all conditions found, the patient's life could be made more tolerable.

Lowther, Macleod and Williamson (1970) offered medical examination to 300 elderly people who lived alone, who had been recently bereaved or who had recently been discharged from hospital. Major conditions were found in 194 patients and recommendations as to therapy or management were carried out in 161 of these. Three per cent of those seen were recommended for admission to hospital. Improvement was found in one-half of the patients who carried out the recommendations; and in 42 per cent of these this improvement was attributed to earlier diagnosis than would have been achieved without the examination at the clinic. Twenty-three per cent of all the patients examined were found, at follow-up 18 to 30 months later, to have been helped by early diagnosis. It was concluded that the offer of a routine examination to a high-risk group of people was of benefit.

Taylor (1972) compared the results of assessment by health visitors in two groups of old people matched for age and social circumstances. One group had been seen by a health visitor six months before the second assessment. Visitors discovered significantly fewer problems requiring attention among the people who had been seen before.

Results of early detection programmes

Early detection programmes help many older people with hearing defect and unsatisfactory sight. Problems with walking are also discovered. Chiropody has to be provided. McLennan et al (1973) showed that 2.4 per cent of elderly people were anaemic. Undiagnosed cardiac failure responds quickly to therapy and hypothyroidism, diagnosed early, is eminently treatable (Bahemuka and Hodkinson, 1975). The haemoglobin level, blood film and electrolytes should be checked, especially when diuretics are being taken.

Agate (1966) has listed the ways in which home accidents can be prevented.

Prevention of mental illness

Depression must be detected while dementia, if diagnosed early, can be assisted by planning for the future. Wilson (1970), a health visitor working among the elderly, felt that social isolation following bereavement could be prevented through support given at the time of greatest grief. The health visitor can overcome loneliness, encourage the intake of an adequate diet and make certain that the elderly person does not become completely cut off from family, friends and neighbours at a time of great risk.

Recommendations for prevention

The Report of an Expert Committee of the World Health Organisation (1974) recommended that:

1. The aged should be considered as a vulnerable group especially susceptible to physical and mental health deterioration and social crises, all of which are closely interrelated. Health surveillance is imperative and demands thorough planning and the organisation of a system of delivery of integrated geriatric services orientated towards keeping the elderly in their own homes and communities wherever possible.
2. Such a system should form an integral part of the general health system and be family and/or community orientated.
3. Each country should assess the unmet needs of the aged and explore the most suitable pattern of care that fits into its health care system, giving special attention to the basic aspects of such a system with its major elements of medical and social prevention, multidisciplinary assessment, home and institutional curative treatment, rehabilitation, long-term care and supportive social welfare.

PRERETIREMENT TRAINING

Some people age successfully by maintaining an active life, while others achieve success through disengagement from their previous level of activity.

The Rutherglen survey revealed few people in the process of voluntarily disengaging from society. Disengagement was due usually to adverse environment or to physical incapacity. In an industrial society in which men and women are educated to work, activity in old age is for many people fundamental to health. This reasoning has resulted in the development of pre- and post-retirement training programmes. The World Health Organisation report (1974) observed that in the developing countries, most people are self-employed and can continue to work as long as they are able; whereas in the developed countries people are generally employed and committed to some form of compulsory retirement that leads to loss of status, reduction of social contacts, decrease in income and financial dependence on the old age pension or a similar source of income.

Leisure activities

Verwoerdt (1976) stated that education towards leisure activities was an essential part of retirement counselling, either pre- or post-retirement.

Since October 1959, over 5000 men and women have taken part in 420 courses for men and 100 for women, organised by the Glasgow Retirement Council. Unanimously, they have expressed appreciation of the courses and have declared themselves as feeling better equipped to plan for their retirement. In the experience of the Glasgow Retirement Council greater benefit is likely to be derived by those who attend a course some two to five years before retirement. The courses are held in colleges for higher education where the older individuals meet the young students and have lunch in the same canteen. Each course consists of an introductory evening meeting followed by seven full-day sessions on one day per week for seven weeks. The employer releases the employee and pays his full salary. The subjects include health in retirement, balancing the budget, mental health, hobbies, e.g. fishing, gardening, appreciation of music and literature, home safety and do-it-yourself repairs to the house. Visits are undertaken to museums, theatres, geriatric units and old people's homes. Every effort is made to instil the belief that retirement is a time of great happiness, of good health and of achievement. Living-in-retirement courses are also held where people who have retired meet together for instruction and guidance.

Re-employment bureaux

The proportion of people in the United Kingdom aged 65 and over who are in employment has fallen sharply, as it has in most economically advanced countries since the beginning of the twentieth century. Approximately one-third of unoccupied old people are willing and able to continue work. Many men of 65 and over feel fit and wish to work, and take most unkindly to society giving them notice that their services are no longer required. In the belief that there will always be some people who desire to work after attaining the age of 65, an office was established in Glasgow in 1967, to arrange part-time paid employment for retired men and women. This office is staffed by retired volunteers, and no charge is made to employees or employers. Between 1967 and 1976 over 1500 retired people were placed in jobs. Men who had held senior executive posts sought positions that would give no worry. Examples of posts obtained are clerical work, handymen, companion-help, bookkeeper, clerks, clerkesses and office managers.

Mutual aid schemes

In the London borough of Merton (Link Opportunity Study, 1975) and elsewhere, schemes have been set up for the exchange of skills among the retired. The giving of a service—whether the expertise of a professional, the skill of a craftsman, the labour of the unskilled or the domestic ability of the housewife, is rewarded by stamps; and these can be used by the recipients to purchase the services they require from the scheme.

Retired employees associations

These consist of people who have worked together in the same industry and who have remained together in retirement. These associations come under the wing of the personnel officers of the firm which employed the older people. Educational activities are provided. Members who are ill are visited by their own colleagues and by the personnel officer.

Hobbies and craft centres

Hobbies and craft centres can be established with the help of the local authority, e.g. in schools. People who have retired can come and make toys or furnishings. Local industrial firms are usually willing to provide machinery. Instruction is given in physical exercise, old-time dancing and topics of the day, while one of the hobbies and craft centres in Glasgow boasts a senior citizens' orchestra.

All-day clubs and lunch clubs

The provision of a cheap but good meal will entice many lonely old people out of their homes. Some old people come together and prepare their own lunches, doing all the cooking themselves, planning menus and washing up afterwards. These clubs can be used to interest older people in keep-fit exercises and dietetic instruction can be given, which is of particular value to widowers.

Telephone reassurance

Help can be given to old people by other elderly persons through daily telephone calls. In some places, elderly invalids in long-term hospitals are taken to telephones and communicate with old people in the same area who live alone, to their mutual benefit.

Friendly visiting

Voluntary visitors take care of one or more old persons and arrange to visit weekly or more often. Street wardens visit daily or twice daily. Training courses for voluntary workers improve their ability to detect early deterioration and inform them about the services available for the elderly in the area. It may be useful to pay an organiser of voluntary work to encourage this type of visiting.

Sheltered housing

In recent years there has been an increase in the demand for warden-supervised houses which allow very frail people to maintain an independent existence out of an institution. Contact with the warden or caretaker is made by an intercommunication system. Many varieties of sheltered housing exist.

Homes for the physically and mentally frail

Some physically and mentally frail elderly can be accommodated in purpose-built homes of about 60 residents with light nursing cover where a therapeutic environment can be created and from where some can then progress to sheltered housing associated with the home.

TV, radio programmes and news-sheets

The elderly greatly appreciate programmes on radio and television and newspapers specially designed for them. Programmes incorporate keep-fit exercises, advice on accident prevention, do-it-yourself techniques, details of pension rights, advice on diet or fashions for the older woman.

Continuing education for the retired

Healthy retired people are a relatively new type. Every effort must be made to accommodate them in a society of which they constitute such a large part. Many older people desire to study in particular a foreign language. Some wish to attend an extramural class or to join classes in the university proper. The older person studying at his own pace can learn almost anything.

PLANNING THE ENVIRONMENT

The immense increase in the number of very old people means that plans must be made now for the creation of an appropriate environment. Students of architecture and town planning, designers of transport and communication and those involved in social work and religious instruction require education in the disabilities and needs of the very old. A report from the United Nations (1975) has a subsection on preventive services to cope with physical deterioration of the environment and environmental hazards. This requests that increased attention must be given to the design and planning of new environments in order to remove architectural hazards and to support older people's physiological, psychological and social capabilities. Physical environments have been created which are hazardous to old people and which fail to support their functional capacities. The report draws attention to the fact that in developed countries the design of communities has been increasingly influenced by the automobile. The construction of highways and traffic patterns has created barriers to the participation of older persons in community life. With the increasing development of new towns and planned communities every attempt should be made to provide physical and psychological environments conducive to permitting older persons to remain active and to have access to community services and resources. The developing countries are reminded of the opportunity to design environments which support activities and needs for the entire life span. Designing environments to support the functional capacities of the ageing is as important as the provision of services and must be a major component of national policy. With appropriate environments within communities as well as within closed settings such as specialised housing and institutions, major problems experienced by the elderly in many parts of the world can be avoided.

WHOSE RESPONSIBILITY?

Elliott and Stevenson (1973) discussed who should care for old people and made the comment that no one in any community should be absolved from responsibility. Professionals have a clear duty in this field, but at a neighbourhood level, the main responsibility must lie with the general practitioner and his team, supported by the geriatric specialist. In addition to his clinical role the geriatrician should be responsible for the continuing education of the general practitioner team and, in collaboration with members of community teams, in the planning of geriatric services in the area. The detail as to who should do the initial medical and social assessment of the elderly should be decided at a local level.

THE FUTURE

The future is bright for preventing or delaying disability in old age. More accurate diagnosis is taking place in the elderly. The word 'senility' is gradually disappearing from acceptable medical terminology, much as did the word 'insanity'. A WHO report (1974) gives a prominent place to prevention in discussing the organisation of geriatric services. The community will benefit from guidance by academic specialists in geriatric medicine, nursing, social work and town and country planning. For too long the sufferings of old people, which are much greater than is often admitted, have been relegated to a 'no-man's land'. Thus the problem has often been dealt with by transferring responsibility from place to place in the hope that it will go away (Rhee, 1974).

Le Gros Clark (1966) stated: 'We understand the category of "employment", and we understand (or believe we understand) the category of "old age". What we have not fully grasped is that technological changes are creating an intermediate stage, often one extending to 10 or 15 years of the life-span. In fact, if we are to have any rational policy in the matter, those who are responsible for our affairs must avoid the fallacy of supposing that the moment at which men are retired from gainful employment is identical with the moment at which old age begins. That is no longer true. . . . Society must be prepared to face up to it.'

REFERENCES

Agate, J. N. (1966) Accidents to old people in their homes. *British Medical Journal*, **ii**, 785.

Akhtar, A. J. (1972) Refusal to participate in a survey of the elderly. *Gerontologia clinica*, **14**, 208.

Akhtar, A. J., Broe, G. A., Crombie, A., McLean, W. M. R., Andrews, G. R. & Caird, F. I. (1973) Disability and dependence in the elderly at home. *Age and Ageing*, **2**, 102.

Anderson, W. F. & Cowan, N. R. (1955) A consultative health centre for older people. *Lancet*, **ii**, 239.

Andrews, G. R., Cowan, N. R. & Anderson, W. F. (1971) The practice of geriatric medicine in the community: an evaluation of the place of health centres. In *Problems and Progress in Medical Care*, Essays on Current Research, 5th Series, ed. McLachlan, G., p. 58. Oxford University Press.

Bahemuka, M. & Hodkinson, H. M. (1975) Screening for hypothyroidism in elderly in-patients. *British Medical Journal*, **ii**, 601.

Barber, J. H. & Wallis, J. B. (1976) Assessment of the elderly in general practice. *Journal of the Royal College of General Practitioners*, **26**, 106.

British Medical Association's Report (1976) *Care of the Elderly*, Report of the Working Party on services for the elderly. BMA House, Tavistock Square, London WC1H 9JP.

Busse, E. W. (1965) The early detection of ageing. *Bulletin of the New York Academy of Medicine*, **41**, 109.

Busse, E. W. (1969) Psychophysiological reactions and psychoneurotic disorders related to physical changes in the elderly. *8th International Congress of Gerontology, Proceedings*, Vol. 1, p. 195. Washington, DC.

Clark, F. le Gros (1966) *Work, Age and Leisure*, p. 151. London: Michael Joseph.

Currie, G. (1975) The care of the elderly. In *General Practice Medicine*, ed. Barber, J. H. & Boddy, F. A. Edinburgh: Churchill Livingstone.

Department of Health and Social Security (1972) A nutrition survey of the elderly. *Report on Health and Social Subjects*, No. 3. London: HMSO.

Elliott, A. E. & Stevenson, J. S. K. (1973) Geriatric care in general practice. *Journal of the Royal College of General Practitioners*, **23**, 615.

Exton-Smith, A. N. & Stanton, B. R. (1965) *Report of an Investigation into the Dietary of Elderly Women Living Alone*. London: King Edward's Hospital Fund.

Gilmore, A. J. J. (1974) Community surveys and mental health. In *Geriatric Medicine*, ed. Anderson, W. F. & Judge, T. G. London: Academic Press.

Hodkinson, H. M., Round, P., Stanton, B. R. & Morgan, C. (1973) Sunlight, vitamin D and osteomalacia in the elderly. *Lancet*, **i**, 910.

Link Opportunity Study (1975) Information from Press Officer, Link Opportunity Study, Flat 6, 40 Shepherd's Hill, London, N.6.

Lowther, C. P., Macleod, R. D. M. & Williamson, J. (1970) Evaluation of early diagnostic services for the elderly. *British Medical Journal*, **iii**, 275–277.
Macleod, C. C., Judge, T. G. & Caird, F. I. (1974a) Nutrition of the elderly at home. I. Intakes of energy, protein, carbohydrate and fat. *Age and Ageing*, **3**, 158.
Macleod, C. C., Judge, T. G. & Caird, F. I. (1974b) Nutrition of the elderly at home. II. Intakes of vitamins. *Age and Ageing*, **3**, 209.
Macleod, C. C., Judge, T. G. & Caird, F. I. (1975) Nutrition of the elderly at home. III. Intake of minerals. *Age and Ageing*, **4**, 49.
Macmillan, D. (1960) Preventive geriatrics. *Lancet*, **ii**, 1439.
Mayer-Gross, W., Slater, E. & Roth, M. (1960) *Clinical Psychiatry*. London: Cassell.
McLennan, W. J., Andrews, G. R., Macleod, C. & Caird, F. I. (1973) Anaemia in the elderly. *Quarterly Journal of Medicine*, **42**, 1.
Milne, J. S., Maule, M. & Williamson, J. (1971) Method of sampling in a study of older people with a comparison of respondents and non-respondents. *British Journal of Preventive and Social Medicine*, **25**, 37.
Pike, L. A. (1969) A screening programme for the elderly in a general practice. *Practitioner*, **203**, 805.
Powell, C. & Crombie, A. (1974) The Kilsyth questionnaire: a method of screening elderly people at home. *Age and Ageing*, **3**, 23.
Rhee, H. A. (1974) *Human ageing and retirement*, pp. 248, 249. Geneva: International Social Security Association.
Ruikka, I. (1971) Geriatrics in Finland. *World Medical Journal*, **18**, 49.
Schwenger, C. W. (1971) Sociomedical care of the aged. *World Medical Journal*, **18**, 42.
Sheldon, J. H. (1948) *The Social Medicine of Old Age*. Oxford University Press.
Stamp, T. C. B. & Round, J. M. (1974) Seasonal changes in human plasma levels of 25-hydroxyvitamin D. *Nature*, **247**, 563.
Stenbäck, A. (1975) Psychosomatic states. In *Modern Perspectives in the Psychiatry of Old Age*, ed. Howells, John G. New York: Brunner/Mazel.
Taylor, B. B. (1972) Personal communication.
Thomas, P. (1968) Experiences of two preventive clinics for the elderly. *British Medical Journal*, **ii**, 357.
United Nations (1975) *The Aging: Trends and Policies*. United Nations Publication. Department of Economic and Social Affairs.
Verwoerdt, A. (1976) *Clinical Geropsychiatry*, Baltimore: Williams & Wilkins Company.
Williams, I. E. (1974) Social background of a group of over 75-year-old patients in general practice. *Gerontologia clinica*, **16**, 203.
Williams, E. I., Bennet, F. M., Nixon, J. V., Nicolson, M. R. & Gabert, J. (1972) Sociomedical study of patients over 75 in general practice. *British Medical Journal*, **ii**, 445.
Williamson, J. (1966) Ageing in modern society. Paper presented to the Royal Society of Health, Edinburgh, 9 November.
Williamson, J., Stokoe, I. H., Gray, S., Fisher, M., Smith, A., McGee, A. & Stephenson, S. (1964) Old people at home: their unreported needs. *Lancet*, **i**, 1117.
Williamson, J., Lowther, C. P. & Gray, S. (1966) The use of health visitors in preventive geriatrics. *Gerontologia clinica*, **8**, 362.
Wilson, F. G. (1970) Social isolation and bereavement. *Lancet*, **ii**, 1356.
World Health Organisation (1974) *Planning and Organisation of Geriatric Services*. Technical Report Series No. 548.

12. Requirement and utilisation of resources by the elderly

M. R. P. Hall

INTRODUCTION

Much research has centred around physical and mental changes in old people as a result of age-associated pathological changes, including the classical studies of Howell (1949), Bedford and Caird (1956), Sheldon (1960) and Newman (1962); the Newcastle studies into the mental health of the elderly (Kay, Beamish and Roth, 1964; Blessed, Tomlinson and Roth, 1968; Kay, Bergmann, Foster, McKechnie and Roth, 1970; Bergmann, 1971; Foster, Kay and Bergmann, 1976); the Scottish studies into the health status of the elderly at home (Williamson, Stokoe, Gray, Fisher, Smith, McGhee and Stephenson, 1964; Andrews, Cowan and Anderson, 1971); studies on the problems of cerebrovascular disease by Adams (1974) in Belfast and Isaacs (1974) in Glasgow; the work of Brocklehurst (1973) on incontinence of urine; and that of Exton-Smith on bedsores (1962), hypothermia (1977), and balance (1977); and the demonstration of the importance of multiple pathology by Wilson and Lawson (1962).

HOSPITAL SERVICES FOR THE ELDERLY

The work done in the United Kingdom by specialist departments of geriatric medicine has increased considerably in recent years. Between 1964 and 1974 the number of beds increased from 54 700 to 55 400; the discharges and deaths per available bed went up from 2.7 to 3.4; and the average length of stay dropped from 129.8 to 98.8 days. Attendance at geriatric outpatient clinics in the same period more than doubled (Social Trends, 1975). The numbers of medical staff increased from 343 to 944 and professorial units were established in nine universities.

Table 1 shows the number of patients aged 65 and over and aged 75 and over who were discharged from or who died in hospitals in England and Wales in 1973. In the country as a whole, 13.7 per cent of the population were aged 65 and over; and of these 35.5 per cent were aged 75 and over. Twenty-one per cent of hospital discharges and deaths were of patients aged 65 and over; but when paediatrics, obstetrics and young chronic sick were excluded this figure rose to 27 per cent. The proportion of hospital beds occupied at any one time by patients aged 65 and over was 49 per cent, compared with 48 per cent in 1972 and 41 per cent in 1968. Over one-third of discharges and deaths from departments of general medicine, chest medicine, ophthalmology, radiotherapy and general practitioner medicine were of patients aged 65 and over (Table 1).

POPULATION PROJECTIONS

According to estimates prepared by the government actuary the number of people in the United Kingdom aged 75 and over will increase by 750 000 by the year 2001; and the number aged 85 years and over will increase by 250 000 by the year 2011. These increases

Table 12.1 Discharges and Deaths from hospitals in the United Kingdom by principal departments to show total all ages, total elderly (65 years and over), and percentage of total elderly who are aged 75 years and over. Source: Hospital Inpatient Enquiry, 1973.

Department	All Ages	Elderly aged 65 years and Over	Percentage of total elderly aged 75 & over
All departments	5 025 290	1 075 930	46
General medicine	724 460	265 840	39.6
Geriatric medicine	200 430	191 890	73
Infectious diseases	45 490	4130	48.9
Diseases of chest	86 170	37 070	33.3
General surgery	993 070	237 510	38.4
Ear, nose and throat	268 280	19 170	32.4
Traumatic & orthopaedic	413 360	91 510	52.1
Ophthalmology	118 680	43 390	47.7
Radiotherapy	43 760	16 700	30.4
Gynaecology	480 840	26 010	28.7
GP other medical	104 430	59 520	58

Table 12.2 Number of beds used daily in hospitals in England and Wales, with proportion occupied by patients aged 65 and over and aged 75 years and over, 1968, 1972 and 1973. Source: Hospital Inpatient Enquiry.

	1968	1972	1973
A. Total (all departments)	199 667	191 963	188 171
B. Total (less paediatrics and obstetrics)	178 330	171 106	168 245
C. Total elderly in geriatric units	47 664	49 828	49 217
Percentage of Total A occupied by elderly (over 65)	43.0	47.8	48.75
Percentage of Total B occupied by elderly (over 65)	48.1	53.7	54.5
Percentage of Total A occupied by over 75's	25.5	29.4	30.1
Percentage of Total B occupied by over 75's	28.5	33.0	33.7
Percentage of Total C occupied by over 75's	73.0	75.9	76.1

indicate the need for greatly expanded services, not only in geriatric medicine, but also in specialties dealing mainly with the elderly, such as orthopaedics and psychiatry.

HOUSING

The general household survey in 1973 showed that 35 per cent of the heads of households in the United Kingdom who were aged 65 and over had lived at their present address for over thirty years; and 39 per cent in this age group occupied accommodation built before 1919. Sixteen per cent of these households lacked a fixed bath, twenty per cent had no internal WC, and 76 per cent were without central heating. Seventy-five per cent of the elderly lived in rooms which did not conform to the Parker-Morris standard for council housing, viz. a minimum temperature of 18.6°C (65°F).

RESIDENTIAL HOMES

The Department of Health and Social Security (HM35/72) suggested that local authorities should provide 25 places per thousand elderly population in residential accommodation, to include three places per thousand for the elderly mental infirm, either in ordinary homes for the elderly or in special homes. Voluntary and private agencies provide a variety of special housing, rest homes and private nursing homes. The amount available depends on the social class and wealth of the local community. In Wessex twenty-five places per thousand elderly were provided by the private sector in the wealthy residential resort of Bournemouth, compared with five in Southampton and three in Portsmouth, which are more industrialised urban areas.

FINANCE

Wroe (1973) found that in 1971 about half the married couples in his sample and a third of the single elderly had incomes above the tax exemption limits, while about 20 per cent of married couples and 33 per cent of single men and 40 per cent of single women received supplementary pensions. Comparatively few elderly households possessed the three major amenities—a telephone, a refrigerator, and a car. (Table 3).

Table 12.3 Some domestic facilities—All households compared to elderly households. Source: General Household Survey.

Domestic Facility	*Percentage in all households*	*Percentage in elderly households*
Telephone	38	27
Refrigerator	69	49
Car	44	20

THE CONCEPT OF NEED

Assessment of need

'Needs' are perceived by observers; 'wants' by the subjects themselves. The evaluation of need may be influenced by the disciplinary bias of the researcher. In a survey carried out by the Danish National Institute of Social Research (Svane, 1971) a random sample of 4200 people aged 70 years and over living in five different areas were asked, among other things, if they wanted a home help or if they wished to enter a nursing home, an old people's home or sheltered housing. The interviewer then made her assessment of the subject's needs; and all subjects who had 'wants' or 'needs' were then re-assessed by their general practitioner and their social worker. Although the provision of home helps varied from 5 per cent of the sample in one area to 25 per cent in another the level of unmet need seemed to be similar. In relation to the need for home help, the interviewer's assessment was highest, followed by the social worker's, then by the elderly person and finally by the doctor. In the case of need for an institution, the highest assessment of need was made by the social worker, followed by the doctor, then by the interviewer and finally by the elderly themselves. These observations reflect the elderly person's desire to remain in his own home, which was supported by the interviewer who was not a health professional. A higher 'need' judged by the health and social services professionals reflected their bias towards institutional care.

Definition of need

Only when 'need' is clearly defined can it be related to the planning of resources, a point discussed by Canvin and Boldy (1976). Research into health and social service provision of the elderly and its use has been undertaken by Harris (1968), and her classical work was followed by many other publications, e.g. Old Age in Hertfordshire (1974); Looking for Trouble Among the Elderly, Coventry Social Services (1973).

The basic needs of the elderly are:

i. Health—to be active and comfortable
ii. Social—to be adequately supported in the community
iii. Occupational—to have a continuing role in society
iv. Spiritual—to be able to continue to develop as an individual.

Geriatric medicine concentrates on the first of these, but recognises that it cannot neglect the others. The geriatrician helps by stimulating the organisational resources in the community through the local authority social services department and voluntary organisations, promoting workshops, employment agencies and educational opportunities.

Meeting need

Table 4 shows the number of professional people available to meet the needs of the elderly in a population of ten thousand. About 95 per cent of the elderly are cared for in their own

Table 12.4 Some key professional personnel available to meet the needs of the elderly in a standard population of 10 000. Source: Wessex Regional Hospital Board.

Consultants:			
General Surgeons	0.15	Social Workers (Hospital)	0.38
General Physicians	0.14	Social Workers (L.A.)	0.8–1.2
General Psychiatrists	0.14	Health Visitors	1.2–1.6
Orthopaedics	0.08	Home Nurses	1.8–2.0
Pathology	0.12	Home Helps	6.3–7.8
Ophthalmologists	0.05		
Geriatricians	0.04		
Local Health Authority MO's	0.53		
General Practitioners	4.00		

homes. Those who cannot be managed at home are referred to other professionals. Two-thirds have complex problems, the solution of which involves large resources, human and material. Recent research has attempted to relate resources to need by endeavouring to measure 'need'.

The behavioural approach to assessing 'need'

It is customary to assess the elderly in terms of activities of daily living (ADL assessment). It is possible to consider elderly patients in 'behavioural' terms and to apply the principles of Behavioural Case Management (Gambriel et al, 1971; Thomas et al, 1971; Thomas and Carter, 1971; and Thomas and Walter, 1973), modified to suit the elderly (Table 12.5). Analysis of performance and goal achievement are essential (Mager and Pipe, 1970; Mager, 1972). The use of problem behaviours as operants, which has helped in the study of abnormal behaviour in children and young adults, may be of value in the elderly (Hoyer et al, 1975).

This approach was used by Kushlick (1976) to plan research into the needs of the elderly, since it makes it possible to quantify observations in relation to need. This led Kushlick's team to look at dependency in terms of help needed by individuals. Those who required support over a period of twelve or twenty-four hours needed the services of a spouse or relative in the home, a residential care attendant in an old people's home, or a nurse in hospital. Isaacs and Neville (1976) used a variation of this method in their study of the measurement of the needs of old people in Scotland. Their subjects were classified into

Table 12.5 Steps necessary in the Management of the elderly patient.

1. Clinical history and examination→data base→problem list
2. Problem selection = mutual agreement between team and patient on problems and priorities
3. Specification of functional capacity necessary to fulfil health need.
4. Baseline assessment i.e. Performance needs against background environment or what is the minimum he has to do at home to achieve A.D.L.
5. Identification of conditions limiting capacity. These may be physical or environmental.
6. Specification of objectives i.e. set goals.
7. (a) Formulate Management (Treatment) Plan
   (b) Implement
   (c) Monitor
8. (a) Formulate maintenance plan
   (b) Implement
   (c) Monitor
9. Discharge
10. Follow up

one of three grades of potential need. The degree of severity depended on the 'interval' elapsing between necessary inputs of help (Table 6). Seven per cent of 419 subjects aged 65–74 years, 14 per cent of 412 subjects in the 75–84 year age group and 37 per cent of those aged 85 years and over had 'critical interval need'. By measuring potential need in this way and comparing it to potential help available Isaacs and Neville were able to estimate met and unmet needs; and by combining three 'potential need' ratings and four 'potential help' ratings they allocated subjects into twelve groups. The total needs of the population studied were then assessed by estimating the services needed to provide the type of help required by each group. This varied from no added service to hospital admission for the most severely disabled. They estimated that the care of 1000 persons aged 65 years or over

Table 12.6 The 'interval' method as a measure of potential need. Source: Isaacs and Neville, 1976.

Grade of severity	*Type of patient and help required*
Long interval need	Help needed at intervals of 24 hrs. or more. Patient can walk indoors, use w.c., boil kettle but unable to do domestic work or shopping
Short interval need	Help needed 2, 3 or 4 times daily. Not capable of making food but can go to w.c.
Critical interval need	Help needed for all activities of daily living. Unable to walk to w.c. and use it without help. Able to be left for short intervals.

required 15 hospital geriatric beds, 10 psychiatric beds, 20 residential home places, 20 home helps, 1 district nurse and 10 'good neighbours', figures similar to those recommended by other surveys (Townsend and Wedderburn, 1965; Harris, 1968 and Hunt, 1970).

Statutory 'norms' of provision

Studies which have clearly indicated the level of provision necessary in order to meet need include those of Townsend and Wedderburn, (1965); Harris (1968); Shanas, Townsend, Wedderburn, Friis, Milhoj and Stehouwer (1968); and the surveys of Hunt (1970) and Marks (1975) of the home help service; and that of Goldberg (1970) of the social work services. As a result of these studies the Department of Health and Social Security advised health authorities and social service departments on the necessary level of services by the publication of 'norms' (Table 7). To achieve these norms would mean increasing available resources in most areas, yet even these norms fall short of those recommended by some research (cf. Isaacs and Neville above).

With the publication of the consultative document 'Priorities for Health and Social Services in England' a first attempt was made to establish rational and systematic priorities throughout the health and personal social services. Yet it is probably wrong to generalise

Table 12.7 Some 'norms' suggested in relation to the elderly.

Social Services Provision (HM 35/72)

Social Work	50/60 per 100 000 total population
Home Helps	12/1000 aged 65 years or more
Mobile meals	200/1000 aged 65 years or more
Day centres	50 places per 100 000 total population
Residential Homes	25 places per 1000 aged 65 years or more

Health Services Provision (DS 329/71 and HM 72/71)
- Hospital beds
  - Medical 10 per 1000 aged 65 years or more
  - Psychiatric 2.5–3 per 1000 aged 65 years or more
  - Medical/Psychiatric Assessment 10–20 per 250 000 total population
- Day Hospital Places
  - Medical 2 per 1000 aged 65 years or more
- Psychiatric 2–3 per 1000 aged 65 years or more.

Housing Provision (No norm for England and Wales)
- Sheltered Housing Places 25/1000 aged 65 years or more (suggested by Scottish Development Department)
  or 50/1000 aged 65 years or more
  (suggested by Townsend (1962)—the Last Refuge. Routledge & Kegan Paul).

with regard to 'norms'. As Gruer (1975) points out in her excellent survey of the Scottish Borders, different interpretations by local authorities of the provision and use of residential homes affect the provision of hospital beds. Similarly, better provision of sheltered housing may alter the need for both residential home and hospital places. Each district or area should develop a policy for the elderly which questions the traditional methods of delivering care. It may be possible to develop 'norms' which relate to the district, allowing the central government to distribute resources more fairly.

Mathematical and strategic considerations

Mathematical solutions are attractive to many planners since they provide a barrier behind which people can hide until the formula has been disproved. Nevertheless they may have their use in relation to a fair distribution of financial resources. Powles (1972) suggested a formula for the allocation of finance which took into account the burden placed on the areas and districts by various health care groups including the elderly. McDonald and his colleagues (1974) developed a mathematical model for the 'balance of care' which was used by Canvin and his colleagues (1976) at the Institute of Biometry and Community Medicine at Exeter University to look at the 'Balance of Care' in Devon and to compare data and assumptions for 1974 and 1981. The 1981 run was used to discover which resource pattern, while maintaining standards, will cost the least. When no limits were put on the expansion of community as opposed to institutional resources, estimated revenue expenditure fell by nearly three million pounds. A third computer run, which aimed at the standards of the consultative document 'Priorities for Health and Personal Social Services' showed an estimated improvement in health services, but social services remained relatively poor.

Cost effectiveness

Little work has been done to assess the cost effectiveness of community care. Wager (1972), comparing residential care and intensive domiciliary care, concluded that there was little difference in cost. Opit (1977) found that in 5 per cent of the patients in his survey who were being cared for at home by a district nurse it was more expensive to provide intensive medical and nursing care at home than it would have been in hospital. The use of limited resources to provide intensive care for some patients at home deprived others of less intensive help.

Health care planning teams

Health Care Planning Teams are multidisciplinary bodies set up under the reorganised National Health Service in the United Kingdom whose function is to advise the district management team on services to the elderly in the district. They consider priorities for the provision of resources to meet need, and develop strategies for planning and monitoring. Canvin and Boldy (1976) suggested a planning framework for the health care planning team to explore priorities; and the South-East Thames Regional Health Authority (1975) undertook a study to identify the information needed to manage health resources used by the elderly. Both these publications emphasised the need to define 'need' and the type of person in need.

CONCLUSION

This review has omitted mention of other areas of need, notably the needs of the deaf, the blind (Brennan and Knox, 1973) and the edentulous (Fish, 1975). In all the areas which have been discussed the important feature is to define and measure 'need' and to relate it to the provision of resources.

REFERENCES

Adams, G. F. (1974) *Cerebrovascular Disability and the Ageing Brain*, Edinburgh: Churchill Livingstone.

Andrews, G. R., Cowan, N. R. & Anderson, W. F. (1971) *Problems and Progress in Medical Care, Essays on Current Research*. 5th Series. ed. McLachlan, G. pp. 58. Oxford: University Press.

Bedford, P. D. & Caird, F. I. (1956) Congestive heart failure in the elderly. *Quarterly Journal of Medicine*, **25**, 407–426.

Bergmann, K. (1971) *The neuroses of old age*. In: Recent Developments in Psychogeriatrics. eds. Kay, D. W. K. & Walk, A. British Journal of Psychiatry Special Publication No. 6, pp. 39–50.

Blessed, G., Tomlinson, B. E. & Roth, M. (1968) The association between quantitative measures of dementia and of senile change in the cerebral grey matter of elderly subjects. *British Journal of Psychiatry*, **114**, 7.

Brennan, M. E. & Knox, E. G. (1973) An investigation into the purposes, accuracy and effectiveness of the Blind Register in England. *British Journal of Preventive & Social Medicine*, **27**, 154–159.

Brocklehurst, J. C. (1973) The Bladder in: *Textbook of Geriatric Medicine & Gerontology*, pp. 298–320. Edinburgh & London: Churchill Livingstone.

British Medical Association (1976) *Care of the Elderly*, Report of the Working Party on Services for the Elderly.

Canvin, R. W. (ed.) (1976) Balance of care in Devon. *Pilot project data and assumptions used for 1974 and 1981 runs of the model.* Institute of Biometry and Community Medicine.

Canvin, R. W. & Boldy, D. P. (1976) *Resource planning within the health care planning teams. Social Science & Medicine*, **10**, 171–176.

Coventry Social Services (1973) *Looking for Trouble Among the Elderly.*

DHSS (1972a) HM35/72 Local Authority Social Services Ten-Year Development Plans, 1973–1993. HMSO: London.

Fish, S. F. (1975) . . . in a good old age, *British Dental Journal*, **138**, 473–479.

Fox, R. H., Woodward, P. M., Exton-Smith, A. N., Green, M. F., Donnison, D. V. & Wicks, M. H. (1973) Body temperatures in the elderly. A national study of physiological, social and environmental conditions. *British Medical Journal*, **1**, 200.

Gambriel, E. D., Thomas, E. J. & Carter, R. D. (1971) Procedure for sociobehavioural practice in open settings. *Social Work*, **16**, 51–62.

Goldberg, E. M. (1970) *Helping the Aged.* National Institute for Social Work Training Series. London: Allen and Unwin Ltd.

Gruer, R. (1975) *Needs of the Elderly in the Scottish Borders.* Scottish Health Service Studies No. 33.

Harris, A. I. (1968) *Social Welfare for the Elderly—Government Social Survey*, Vol. II. London: HMSO.

Howell, T. H. (1949) Senile deterioration of the central nervous system, *British Medical Journal*, **i**, 56–58.

Hoyer, W. J., Mishara, B. L. & Riebel, R. G. (1975) Problem behaviours as operants. *The Gerontologist*, **15**, 452–456.

Hunt, A. (1970) The home help service in England and Wales, HMSO: London.

Isaacs, B. (1974) *Survival of the Unfittest*, Studies of Illness and Death in the Elderly in Glasgow, Scottish Health Service Study No. 17, Scottish Home & Health Department.

Isaacs, B. & Neville, Y. (1976a) The Measurement of Need in Old People, *Scottish Health Service Studies*, No. 34.

Isaacs, B. & Neville, Y. (1976b) The needs of old people: the 'interval' as a method of measurement. *British Journal of Preventive and Social Medicine*, **30**, 79–85.

Kay, D. W. K., Bergmann, K., Foster, E. M., McKohnie, A. A. & Roth, M. (1970) Mental illness and hospital usage in the elderly: a random sample followed up. *Comp. Psychiatry*, **11**, 26–35.

Kay, D. W. K., Beamish, P. & Roth, M. (1964) Old age mental disorders in Newcastle upon Tyne, Part I: A study of prevalence, *British Journal of Psychiatry*, **110**, 146–158.

Kushlick, A., Felce, D., Palmer, J. & Smith, J. (1976) Evidence to the Committee of Inquiry into mental handicap nursing and care from the Health Care Evaluation Team, Winchester—*Research Report* Wessex Regional Health Authority.

Mager, R. E. & Pipe, P. (1970) *Analyzing Performance Problems.* Belmont, California: Fearon.

Mager, R. E. (1972) *Goal Analysis.* Belmont, California: Lear Sergler/Fearon.

Marks, J. (1975) Home Help—a study of needs, management and home help staff in a local authority. *Occasional Papers on Social Administration* No. 58. London: Bell and Sons.

McDonald, A. G., Cuddeford, G. C. & Beale, E. M. L. (1974) Balance of Care: some mathematical models of the National Health Service. *British Medical Bulletin*, **30**, 262–271.

Newman, J. L. (1962) Old folk in wet beds. *British Medical Journal*, **1**, 1824–1827.

Norton, D., McLaren, R. & Exton-Smith, A. N. (1962) *An investigation of Geriatric Nursing Problems in Hospital*, National Corporation for the Care of Old People. London: Nuffield Foundation.

Opit, L. J. (1977) Domiciliary care for the elderly sick—economy or neglect ? *British Medical Journal*, **1**, 30–33.

Overstall, P. W., Exton-Smith, A. N., Imms, F. J., Johnson, A. L. (1977) Falls in the elderly related to postural imbalance. *British Medical Journal*, **1**, 261–264.

Powles, J. (1972) quoted in 'Care of the Elderly' Wessex Regional Hospital Board.

Shanas, E., Townsend, P., Wedderburn, D., Friis, H., Milhoj, P. & Stehouwer, J. (1968) *Old People in Three Industrial Societies*, London: Routledge & Kegan Paul.

Sheldon, J. H. (1960) Problems of an ageing population. *British Medical Journal*, **2**, 1223–1235.

Svane, O. (1971) *Assessment of Needs of Care for the Elderly.* The National Institute of Social Research, Copenhagen.

Thomas, E. J. & Carter, R. D. (1971) Instigative modification with a multi-problem family. *Social Case Work*, **52**, 444–455.

Thomas, E. J., Abrams, K. S. & Johnson, J. B. (1971) Self-monitoring and reciprocal inhibition in the modification of multiple tics of Gilles de la Tourette's syndrome. *Journal of Behaviour Therapy and Experimental Psychiatry*, **2**, 159–171.

Thomas, E. J. & Walter, C. L. (1973) Guidelines for behaviour practice in the open community agency: procedure and evaluation. *Behaviour Research and Therapy*, **11**, 193–205.

Thompson, E. J. (ed.) (1975) *Social Trends, No. 6*, Central Statistical Office, London: HMSO.
Townsend, P. & Wedderburn, D. (1965) *The Aged in the Welfare State*, London: Bell & Sons Ltd.
Wager, R. (1972) *Care of the Elderly*—an exercise in Cost Benefit Analysis. London: Institute of Municipal Treasurers and Accountants.
Wessex Regional Hospital Board (1972) *Care of the Elderly*: Report of a Working Party, Vol. 3.
Williamson, J., Stokoe, I. H., Gray, S., Fisher, M., Smith, A., McGhee, A. & Stephenson, E. (1964) Old People at home—their unreported need, *Lancet*, **i**, 1117–1120.
Wilson, L. A., Lawson, I. R. & Brass, W. (1962) Multiple disorders in the elderly. A clinical and statistical study. *Lancet*, **ii**, 841–843.
Wroe, D. C. L. (1973) The Elderly, *Social Trends No. 4*, ed. Missel, M., Central Statistical Office, London: HMSO.

Index